pandexicon / (pandemic + lexicon)

1. *A lexicon of the pandemic.*
2. *A collection of short essays related to words and phrases particular to the Covid-19 pandemic.*

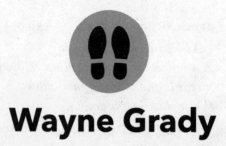

Wayne Grady

pan·dex·i·con

/ pan-ˈdek-sə-kän / *n.*

How the Language of the Pandemic
Defined Our New Cultural Reality

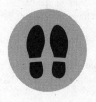

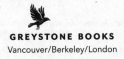

GREYSTONE BOOKS
Vancouver/Berkeley/London

Greystone Books Ltd.
greystonebooks.com

Cataloguing data available from Library and Archives Canada
ISBN 978-1-77840-039-1 (cloth)
ISBN 978-1-77840-040-7 (epub)

Editing by Nancy Flight
Copy editing by James Penco
Proofreading by Dawn Loewen
Cover and text design by Jessica Sullivan

Printed and bound in Canada on FSC® certified paper
at Friesens. The FSC® label means that materials used for
the product have been responsibly sourced.

Greystone Books thanks the Canada Council for the Arts, the
British Columbia Arts Council, the Province of British Columbia
through the Book Publishing Tax Credit, and the Government
of Canada for supporting our publishing activities.

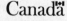

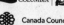

MIX
Paper from
responsible sources
FSC® C016245

BRITISH COLUMBIA

BRITISH COLUMBIA ARTS COUNCIL
An agency of the Province of British Columbia

Canada Council   Conseil des arts
for the Arts   du Canada

Greystone Books gratefully acknowledges the xʷməθkʷəy̓əm (Musqueam), Sḵwx̱wú7mesh (Squamish), and səlílwətaʔɬ (Tsleil-Waututh) peoples on whose land our Vancouver head office is located.

Contents

Introduction:
A Few Words

WHEN COUNTRIES STARTED closing their borders, my wife and I were in Mexico. There are many stories like ours. It was late March 2020; we heard from people who were stranded in England or Portugal or Australia. There was a scramble to get home. Someone fell and broke her hip; someone else decided they'd rather stay in Spain. We managed to get seats on the last flight out of Mexico City before the airline cut its schedule to once a week. We bought business-class tickets because we wanted to get on the plane last and off first. We thought it would be safer—no milling around in crowded aisles—but we weren't sure. In any case, the airplane sat on the runway for three hours with the door open while we waited for a mechanic to repair a ventilator fan. When we finally arrived in Toronto, fourteen hours after leaving San Miguel de Allende, we were herded through customs at the same time as hundreds of people who'd been on a flight from New York—with no social distancing and very few face masks.

In Canada, two hundred people had already died of Covid-19. We thought that was a lot. We had booked a connecting flight to Kingston, Ontario, where we live, but we were already thinking of airplanes as flying incubators, so we rented a car instead. When we stopped for gas, we paid at the pump. We arrived home at three in the morning, exhausted, confused, worried that we'd brought something with us from Mexico, picked something up on the plane, caught something at the airport. Everything familiar was suddenly a threat.

And that was the beginning.

ILLNESS CHANGES EVERYTHING. Natural disasters tend to make us mistrust nature. Human-caused calamities make us mistrust each other. During a pandemic, which is both natural and human-spread, we mistrust everything. Including ourselves. For all of our adaptability, our species doesn't like change, and we respond especially badly to rapid change. As soon as we can, we employ our much-vaunted ingenuity to make our new surroundings familiar, and one of the ways we do that is through language. When we come up with a new word or adapt an existing phrase to describe the new phenomenon—a war, a school of thought, a pandemic—we are domesticating change, taking the threat out of it. We don't say that during the war we bombed hospitals; we say we defended democracy and invented the ballpoint pen.

How can we harbor bad memories of a war that gave us Spam and the jeep? After the Middle Ages, the misery of the Black Death—which wiped out half of Europe and a third of the Middle East in the fourteenth century, and surged again in the seventeenth—faded when we began using "plague" to describe any minor annoyance. As in Philip Larkin's novel *A Girl in Winter*, when the main character complains that "the pipes aren't hot. They never are," another replies, "It's a plague." Or when Ottessa Moshfegh writes, in the *New Yorker*, that whether she was "drinking at a bar or alone at home, self-centered dissatisfaction plagued me." Percy Bysshe Shelley employed the term "pandemic" to mean something like "carnal": "That Pandemic lover who loves rather the body than the soul, is worthless." When illness sounds more like everyday language, it ceases to be a disaster and becomes the new normal.

As Susan Sontag writes in *Illness as Metaphor*, "The very names of... diseases are felt to have a magic power." And so we avoid using them. On countless tweets and TikToks, the word "pandemic" became the "Panda Express," or the "panini," or the "Pandora," or the "Panasonic." No one worried about a panda or was vaccinated against panini bread. We were safe. We didn't say "a vaccination"; we called it a shot (in the US), or a jab (in the UK and Australia). "Quarantine" was drawled into "cornteen"; what could be more common than corn? "Coronavirus" became "the Rona" or "Miss Rona," the slightly wild woman who lives on a dark street at the edge of town. A friend writing about Omicron called it "the Omigod variant." In Sweden, Covid-19 was called "the Corona," which means "crown," or *kronor* in Swedish, which is that country's currency and national emblem. In the US, when it was mostly eighty-year-olds who were dying, Covid-19 was known as "the Boomer Remover"—more sinister than Miss Rona, but still funny.

Humorous euphemisms allow us to talk about what frightens us without wallowing in morbidity; we can discuss the pandemic without having to think about it. For a time. When people in their twenties started dying, no one called it "the Zoomer Remover"; the disease reverted to being Covid-19, or more familiarly, Covid. As the body count rose, jokes became hollow. We switched back to calling the crisis what it was, because the pandemic had become more familiar to us than the euphemisms.

"By being able to talk about the crisis," says Christine Möhrs, a linguist at the Leibniz Institute for the German Language, "we reduce our fears. We can share our insecurities." Germans created more than 1,200 new words with which to talk about the pandemic, from *Ausgangsbeschränkung* (going-out restriction, or lockdown) to *Anderthalb-Meter-Gesellschaft* (one-and-a-half-meter society, or social distancing). France introduced the term *quatorzaine* to refer to the fourteen-day isolation period after exposure to the virus, and in the Netherlands, the frantic hoarding of groceries was called *hamsteren*—hamstering. We hamstered items we thought would soon be in short supply. Families hamstered batteries, toilet paper, and coffee; countries hamstered vaccine doses.

Around the world, the pandemic brought aspects of our lives to light in new ways. Handwashing, an act ordinarily performed without thinking, became a conscious, specific procedure complete with precise instructions. In China, schoolchildren made hats with ninety-centimeter brims; when two brims touched, the wearers were socially distanced. In Canada, a face mask was no longer something hockey dads bought at Canadian Tire; it became "PPE" (personal protective equipment), something the country's chief medical officer urged everyone to wear in public.

Cloth face masks have become fashion accessories and even collectible art objects. Our friend in San Miguel, Lena Bartula, an American fabric artist who owns an art gallery there, created beautiful oversized *cubrebocas*—mouth-covers, the new Spanish word for face masks—which she wore and also mounted on the wall above her Mexican *huipils*. She called them "artifacts from the time in between." When life deals us lemons, we use them to make art.

And like art, a pandemic alters the way we think about ourselves and each other. The day after we returned from Mexico, a neighbor who was making cloth masks for her family and friends gave us two.

There were instructions on YouTube for making face masks out of old T-shirts, but our neighbor's masks were things of beauty. They had white fabric linings, pipe cleaners sewn in to bend over the nose, and elastic ear loops. There was a dark, roses-on-black pattern for me and a lighter, forget-me-not one for my wife, Merilyn. Our university town wasn't locked down yet, but face masks and social distancing were strongly recommended, and stores were limiting the number of customers allowed in at a time. We walked downtown with our masks on, feeling protected but a little self-conscious; mine was a bit small and made my ears stick out. Our glasses steamed up. My nose became stuffed and runny. Not everyone we saw was wearing a mask, and some of those who were had pulled them down below their noses; others had them under chins so they could smoke or drink take-out coffee. Restaurant patios were still open, but not to capacity. Groups of young people passed us, yelling and carrying on in a way that was likely to spray globules of virus-laden moisture everywhere. They seemed oblivious to what was going on in the world around them. Or perhaps they were making a statement, we thought—town and gown, us and them, timid compliers and youthful rebels. They probably weren't saying to themselves that they didn't care if we died. But they were behaving that way.

Some of that divisive thinking will remain with us, just as some Covid variant will very likely always be a source of concern, and the new vocabulary will remain in the language as connotations, if not as denotations, of our collective ordeal. We have always patted our pockets when leaving the house—first it was for wallet and keys; then it was for wallet, keys, and phone; now it's for wallet, keys, phone, and face mask. When the Covid crisis is over, if it is ever over, we will still check our pockets for face masks when we go out or find an old N95 crumpled up in a hall table drawer and think, "Oh, yes, I remember those days." When we see a group of people standing together in a park, we will count them, and notice how far apart they are keeping. Like ballpoint pens and Spam, our new habits will persist into the After Times, just as, after the First World War, no veteran lit three cigarettes with a single match. In 2020, I watched in sympathy and horror as protesters across the US gathered to commemorate the murder of George Floyd, but part of me was thinking, "They aren't social distancing."

New phrases entered our daily vocabularies: self-isolation, community spread, social distancing. A person with a disease, writes Virginia Woolf in "On Being Ill," is confronted with the poverty of the language to convey the immensity of their sickness, and is "forced to coin words himself, and, taking his pain in one hand, and a lump of pure sound in the other... so to crush them together that a brand-new word in the end drops out." She adds that the new word will probably "be something laughable." And so we invented "hydroxymoron," "coronnial," and "Covexit."

Terminology that had formerly been used by health professionals—"immunocompromised," "underlying health conditions"—began showing up in newspaper headlines. Old familiar phrases took on new and sinister dimensions. Companies that didn't "pivot" didn't survive. Variants caused an "uptick" in cases. I'm guessing that after Covid-19, families will think a long time before putting their elderly parents in long-term care facilities.

I have gathered, in this book, some of the terms that kept appearing in newspapers and online pandemic coverage to form a kind of lexicon of our shared experience. I have omitted most catchwords, like "the Rona," "maskne" (the skin condition that frontline workers got from wearing face masks for twelve hours a day), and "covidiot" (someone who refuses to take precautions against being infected or infecting others). Such terms flared up in the fevered darkness of our coronaviral night, illuminated a moment or a scene, and faded again into obscurity when the situation that gave them a stage moved on to other theatres. "The Rona" appeared for a few weeks and then disappeared from use. And "maskne" cleared up with a bit of antiseptic cream; with patients dying around them, no one complained about blemishes behind their ears. "Covidiot" gave way to "anti-masker" and "anti-vaxxer," which were less funny but more descriptive. I have tried to keep to words that will live on, as "jeep" and "apocalypse" are still with us from previous disasters. Will temporary disorientation now be referred to as "brain fog"? Will we describe the sky above Mexico as being "face-mask blue"?

In contrast to other lexicons, I have not arranged the words alphabetically. By grouping together words and phrases that seem to me to be related—all the "cures" for Covid to which people turned in panic, for example—I have tried to make a narrative history of the pandemic rather than an alphabetized account. And I have further arranged these groupings into chapters, in an attempt to convey a sense of the chronology, from the Before Times to the much-hoped-for After Times, in a way that distantly echoes the division of the pandemic into successive waves comprising distinct variants. Like the pandemic, the structure of this book is organic.

THE PANDEMIC HAS entered our language—and languages around the world—as it has entered our lives. It is both pandemic and pandemonium, the corruption of our lungs and of our social fabric. It has been a psychological as much as a physiological ordeal. We have turned to Zoom and FaceTime for human contact, platforms that were devised as alternatives to human contact. We have executed gymnastic arabesques to stay six feet from passersby on narrow sidewalks; surely social distancing should have been called anti-social distancing. We've noticed when someone didn't follow the arrows or stand on the footprints painted on the floors of supermarkets. We've denied entrance to people who came to the door unmasked. We have been vexed when the bottle of hand sanitizer at the drugstore entrance was empty or its foot pedal was broken. We have sympathized with, or counted ourselves among, the thousands of employees who lost their jobs when businesses closed, but at the same time wondered if we'd ever again feel comfortable in a crowded office or restaurant.

"We yearned for the future," Offred recalls in Margaret Atwood's *The Handmaid's Tale*, looking back to "the time before." We, too, yearn for the future: we call it the After Times, and, like Offred, we aren't really sure it will come.

1

The Before Times

"In rich nations such as the United States, infectious diseases are mostly relatively minor causes of death, but there is no guarantee that situation will continue." PAUL AND ANNE EHRLICH, *Betrayal of Science and Reason*, 1996

Before Times / *The fondly remembered halcyon days before the pandemic.*

The pandemic has distorted the mirror of time for all of us; we feel time differently. How long have we been self-isolating? Was the second wave in the fall of 2020 or the winter of 2021? Was it last March when the airports were empty, or the March before that? The days are slow, the waiting seems endless, and yet we can't recall in any detail what we did. Every day of the pandemic is like a day spent in a dying loved one's hospital room.

Marina Koren, writing in *The Atlantic*, catches the whimsicality of looking back to better days. During the pandemic, she writes, we've had to grapple with the sense "that the days before the coronavirus swept across the country—the 'Before Time,' as many have been calling it—feel like a bygone era." She observes that behavior that seemed mundane before the pandemic—shaking hands, touching our uncovered faces, standing close to others in a group—can trigger sudden, visceral reactions; an act of kindness, a peck on the cheek, a brief hug, are now seen as reckless acts that can spread disease. "It almost seems," Koren writes, "as if the response to the pandemic has somehow, quietly and without warning, rewired our brains." When we think of the things we did in the Before Times we feel ourselves to have been quaintly naive, if not mindlessly dangerous. It's like remembering someone running with scissors.

The word "beforetime," in the King James Version of the Bible, means more than simply "in the past." It means in a better time, more like "in the good old days." Except that the pandemic isn't yet a time that has passed; we are still living in the midst of an apocalyptic rupture. The Grim Reaper's scythe is still whistling past our heads. The *Wall Street Journal* writer Ben Zimmer traces the modern origin of the phrase to a 1966 *Star Trek* episode in which Captain Kirk and Spock land on a planet peopled solely by children who have survived a human-made plague (and one that, at least at first, didn't affect children). An experiment conducted by grown-ups went disastrously wrong, and one of the children says, "That was when they started to get sick in the Before Time."

That a pandemic that blurs and distorts our sense of time invokes phrases from science fiction isn't surprising. I am reminded of a 1971 novel by Ursula K. Le Guin, *The Lathe of Heaven*, which takes place in Portland, Oregon, in 2002, which was then the not-so-distant future. George Orr has a problem: everything he dreams comes true, but not in the way he wanted. (Perhaps George Orr is George Orwell with the "well" removed.) When Orr dreams of a world without racism, he wakes up to find that everyone has gray skin. And when he dreams of a world that is not overpopulated, he awakens to a reality in which a mysterious plague has killed most of the humans on Earth. Le Guin was a brilliant, complex, and highly imaginative novelist, and *The Lathe of Heaven* explores the danger of tinkering with the mind, especially since what we call "reality" may simply be a figment of our own imaginations. The future certainly is.

There is, however, a simpler lesson to be taken from the novel: if you long for the Before Times—or worse, behave as though the Before Times were still with us—you could die.

Zoonosis / *An infectious disease of animals that is communicable to humans.*

Zoonotic diseases challenge the notion that humans are somehow different from animals. Humans contract infectious diseases from animals with alarming frequency, and such "spillover" diseases often become pandemic. As David Quammen writes in *Spillover*, "the subject of animal disease and the subject of human disease are... strands of one braided cord." And zoonotic diseases are becoming ever more frequent as humans come into closer contact with wild animals. As we turn more wilderness into agricultural land and poach more wild game for human consumption—both in the interests of feeding our ever-growing population—we run the risk of picking up more and more diseases from the wild animals we encounter.

Of the more than 1,400 pathogens that human flesh is heir to, 60 percent originated in animals, usually other vertebrates. In a sense, then, we are paying the price for our domestication of animal species that began 18,000 years ago, when humans domesticated cassowaries for food. Avian influenza (H5N1), which broke out in numerous places in 1997, found a convenient replication machine in the world's burgeoning chicken factories; Lyme disease enters human pathways via ticks, often transferred to humans by domestic dogs and cats; rabies also spills over to us from wild canines and raccoons by means of dogs; and mad cow disease made its way from cattle to humans after farmers began feeding infected meat-and-bone meal to their livestock.

The seven types of coronaviruses that affect humans originate in either bats or birds. The coronavirus that caused the SARS-COV-1 outbreak at first infected leaf-nosed bats (family Phyllostomidae), then spread to horseshoe bats (Rhinolophidae), then to Asian palm civets (*Paradoxurus hermaphroditus*)— furry, arboreal animals that look like cats and are sold in Asian markets for food, which is how the virus eventually spilled over to humans. The coronavirus that causes Covid-19 is a new strain of betacoronavirus, also originating in bats, that is 79 percent similar to the SARS-COV-1 virus and is suspected to have reached humans along a similar pathway, although instead of palm civets, the transition host between bats and humans for Covid is thought to have been pangolins (of *Manis* spp.), armored anteaters from Asia. Pangolins are the most poached and illegally trafficked animals in the world—all eight species (four Asian and four African) are endangered. The biggest market for these animals is China, where they are sold for food as well as for use in traditional medicine. They turn up in live-animal wet markets such as the one in Wuhan, the city in central China where Covid-19 was first detected.

It's not certain that pangolins were the bridge species between bats and humans. Just as no bat with the Covid virus has been found, so no pangolin with Covid has come to light. But a study conducted by the Francis Crick Institute, published in February 2021 in *Nature Communications*, found that proteins in the Covid coronavirus were similar to those in a coronavirus isolated from Malayan pangolins smuggled into China, which suggests not only that the virus could have spilled over directly from pangolins to humans but also that the Covid outbreak in Wuhan—in effect, the entire ensuing pandemic—may have been the result of the illegal trafficking of pangolins into China. Donald Benton, the co-lead author of the study, apparently drew that inference: although the study found no direct evidence "to prove definitively that this virus did pass through pangolins to humans," he wrote, "we have shown that a pangolin virus could potentially jump to humans, so we urge caution in any contact with this species and the end of illegal smuggling and trade in pangolins."

Andrew Nikiforuk, in his book *Pandemonium* (2006) about the spread of zoonotic diseases, argues pandemics are the logical outcome of globalization. "Ultimately," he writes, "a severe pandemic might encourage us to rethink the deadly pace of globalization and biological traffic in all living things."

"Maybe," he adds, "we will learn that we can't liberalize trade without liberating biology in unpredictable ways."

Coronavirus / *A positive-strand* RNA *virus causing mild to severe respiratory illness in several animals, including cows, bats, and humans. (A positive-strand* RNA *virus is one whose genetic material functions both as genome and as messenger* RNA, *which means it can translate more directly into viral protein in the host cell and thus replicate itself more quickly than other types of viruses.)*

A virus is an odd life-form. The word derives from the Latin for "poison" and originally referred to noxious bodily secretions, such as pus. Biologically, a virus is simply a package of nucleic acids—the primary information-carrying molecules in all cells and viruses—encased in a protein shell. When a virus enters a host, its shell dissolves, exposing its genes, which instruct the host's internal machinery to replicate the virus rather than the host's own cells. A virus is not, by itself, a living organism—unlike a bacterium, it doesn't "live" until it has invaded a host and co-opted its software. And yet, before doing so, it is not "dead." Luis P. Villarreal, writing in *Scientific American* (August 8, 2008), says that because viruses are composed of the same building blocks as true life-forms, they are, though not fully alive, "more than inert matter: they verge on life."

The family of viruses to which SARS-COV-2 belongs was first captured on an electron micrograph in 1965 by June Almeida, a Scottish lab technician working at St. Thomas's Hospital Medical School in London. Earlier, while working as an electron microscope technician at the Ontario Cancer Institute in Canada, she had perfected a method of imaging viruses by staining them with phosphotungstic acid—a common dye used to make viruses, nerves, and other organic material visible under electron microscopes. Using this method, she discovered a viruslike particle in cancer patients' blood.

In 1964, Almeida was lured back to the UK to work at St. Thomas's by Dr. David Tyrrell, who wanted images of the viruses he was researching that caused the common cold. There, she micrographed a new type of coronavirus that Tyrrell had been unable to replicate in the lab. The image she produced showed a virus consisting of a central nucleus surrounded by a series of antenna-like protein spikes with strange protuberances at their tips; Almeida, Tyrrell, and Tony Waterson, a professor of medical microbiology at St. Thomas's, named the unknown virus a "coronavirus" because the protuberances reminded them of crowns.

Of the seven known types of coronaviruses that have spilled over from their animal hosts to humans, four cause the common cold, two others caused the SARS and Middle East respiratory syndrome (MERS) epidemics, and the seventh is the latest new, or novel, coronavirus that has given us Covid-19. The scientific name of this coronavirus is SARS-CoV-2, sometimes shortened to SARS-2. It's the virus that has made us all feel we are verging on life.

While she was at the Ontario Cancer Institute, June Almeida composed a poem, à la William Blake, expressing her fascination with her subject and with the microbiological world in which she worked:

> Virus, Virus shining bright,
> In the phosphotungstic night,
> What immortal hand or eye,
> Dare frame thy fivefold symmetry.

SARS-COV-2 / *Severe acute respiratory syndrome coronavirus 2, the strain of coronavirus that causes Covid-19. So called to distinguish it from SARS-COV-1, the strain that caused the SARS outbreak in 2003.*

The Covid-19 coronavirus was originally referred to by some as "the Wuhan coronavirus," or "the Wuhan virus," because it was first detected in that city in central China in December 2019. In January 2020, the World Health Organization (WHO) recommended it be termed "2019 novel coronavirus," or 2019-nCov, in accordance with the WHO's 2015 guideline against using geographic locations, animal species, or groups of people when naming a disease (as in "swine flu" and "Spanish flu"). Such use, said one WHO official, could "provoke a backlash against members of particular religious or ethnic communities," as had happened in 1918, when the influenza that killed 50 million people in eighteen months was called the Spanish flu. In the US, because of the name of the disease, immigrants from Latin America were subjected to racism and social stigma, presumably because they spoke Spanish.

The official name for the disease, "coronavirus disease 2019," later shortened to Covid-19, was adopted on February 11, 2020, by the International Committee on Taxonomy of Viruses (ICTV). And yet, in a tweet on March 16, then US president Donald Trump still referred to it as the "Chinese virus" and repeated the term often in interviews and press briefings. He seemed to take an adolescent's delight in defying the WHO and vilifying the Chinese. "China," he said, "tried to say, at one point—maybe they stopped now— that it was caused by American soldiers. That can't happen." (China did post messages on Facebook and Twitter saying the US Army had engineered Covid-19.)

Trump pretended to stop calling Covid-19 "the Chinese flu" later in March, saying "nasty language" was being used against Asian Americans. There was more than nasty language; according to the American Psychological Association (APA), hate incidents against Asian Americans and Pacific Islanders doubled during the pandemic, from 3,795 in March 2020 to 6,603 by March 2021, and included "episodes rang[ing] from verbal harassment, insults, and jokes … to violent attacks in schools, businesses, and other public spaces." But Trump and his associates continued to use anti-Asian slurs. On March 25, 2020, when G7 foreign ministers met online to discuss their responses to the pandemic, they failed to come to an agreement on a joint statement, because then US secretary of state Mike Pompeo insisted on referring to "the Wuhan virus." And in June, Trump amused a crowd at a campaign rally in Tulsa, Oklahoma, by referring to Covid-19 as "kung flu."

It's true that we continue to use geographic or animal names for many infectious diseases that affect humans. We still refer to Ebola (a river in the Democratic Republic of the Congo) and Zika (a forest in Uganda), the Marburg virus (Marburg is a town in Germany), Middle East respiratory syndrome (MERS), and Hendra virus (a suburb of Brisbane, Australia). But we don't do so to incite hatred and violence. No one hates chickens because of chicken pox. Trump and his staff knew exactly what they were doing when they referred to Covid-19 as "the China virus." They were invoking a sense of dread and danger, echoing the 1979 disaster movie *The China Syndrome*, about a meltdown at a nuclear power plant (ironically, the fictional power plant was in the US and had nothing whatever to do with China.)

Even when Trump was ostensibly telling his followers not to use the term, he was planting the words in the minds of people already inclined to racism. He was using the rhetorical device employed by Br'er Rabbit in the Uncle Remus stories: Br'er Rabbit keeps saying, "Please don't throw me into that briar patch," when in fact he wants nothing more than to be thrown into the briar patch. Likewise, Trump was covertly telling his followers to blame the pandemic on the Chinese. He gave the same kind of covert message to the white supremacist group the Proud Boys, when he told them to "stand back and stand by."

Jack Wang, author of *We Two Alone*, a collection of stories about the Chinese diaspora, noted that "the President and his minions were doubling and tripling down on the phrase 'the China virus.' This kind of rhetoric has led to a well-documented spike in vitriol and violence against those of Asian descent, not just in the US but the world over, including Canada. People yelled at, spat on, pushed and shoved, kicked and punched, chased through the street. More harrowing still, slashed across the face with a knife while shopping, doused with acid while taking out the trash." In one tragic example of this bigotry, on March 16, 2021, a man named Robert Aaron Long targeted Asian women at three health spas in Atlanta, Georgia, killing eight people.

Scientifically, when it first started going viral, SARS-CoV-2 presented a number of traits that confused epidemiologists. For one thing, researchers didn't know why the virus, before its many mutations, seemed to have little effect on children: those under the age of about five could have been infected with SARS-CoV-2 without showing clinical signs of Covid-19.

This was reminiscent of AIDS research, during which thousands of chimpanzees were injected with HIV, but in ten years only about a hundred of them developed AIDS. Another puzzle was the variety of ways Covid-19 affected those who did get it. Some developed Covid-19 but didn't know they had it, others came down with mild symptoms that lasted a few days, others remained seriously ill for months on end—the so-called long-haulers—and still others died from it. Altogether, researchers have recorded nearly two hundred symptoms related to Covid-19.

Another aspect of SARS-COV-2 that makes it dangerous is the way it behaves once it enters our bodies. Most viruses, when they encounter a host cell, replace about 10 percent of that cell's genetic makeup with their own; SARS-COV-2 replaces 60 percent. When a host cell is invaded, it usually does two things: emits interferons to alert neighboring cells that an invasion has taken place, and then sends cytokines to the body's immune system to get it to start manufacturing white blood cells, which then produce antibodies to fight off the invasion.

Most viruses shut down both of those responses so that the virus can spread to other cells unimpeded. But SARS-COV-2 behaves differently: it stops the invaded cell from alerting its neighbors so that the virus can spread quickly over a large area, but it allows the invaded cells to send cytokines to kick-start the immune system. With so many infected cells sending out alarm signals at once, the infected area is flooded with white blood cells in a "cytokine storm," thereby clogging the body's circulatory system with antibodies. Most of these antibodies are not specific against the coronavirus; they just begin attacking everything in their path.

"As they do their work," James Somers writes in the November 9, 2020, issue of the *New Yorker*, "inflammation distends the lungs, and debris fills them like a fog." A person with Covid-19 strongly resembles a patient with an autoimmune disorder: the body manufactures so many antibodies that it begins attacking itself. Left untreated, the cytokine storm clogs the patient's lungs, the patient develops severe hypoxia—or lack of oxygen in the blood—and dies. This is why a reliable oxygen supply is crucial in hospitals inundated with Covid patients. Throughout the pandemic, almost half the patients whose cases of Covid proved fatal died from lack of oxygen.

Researchers at the University of Alberta, led by Dr. Shokrollah Elahi, found that when blood oxygen levels diminish, the body begins to manufacture immature red blood cells, which do not transport oxygen; only mature red blood cells do. Furthermore, immature red blood cells are highly susceptible to viral infection. Dr. Elahi and his colleagues showed that immature red blood cells express the receptor ACE2, which is precisely the receptor to which the spike proteins on a coronavirus attach when it encounters a human cell. The more ACE2 receptors we have, the more readily a coronavirus will enter our cells.

Much of the initial confusion about the nature of SARS-CoV-2 was the result of the swiftness with which it spread. Chinese virologists published the virus's genome on January 11, 2020 (before the Chinese government shut down their lab), and researchers around the world scrambled to comprehend the blatant beast they were facing. Then, just as they were close to understanding one form of Covid, the coronavirus would mutate and create a variant that behaved in a startlingly different manner from its predecessor. But as time passed and more researchers became involved in Covid-19 studies, the complicated nature of the virus became more evident. Eighteen months into the pandemic, for example, *The Guardian* published an update explaining what health authorities knew about Covid then that they hadn't known before, such as the significance of aerosol transmission (and therefore the importance of wearing face masks), the role of asymptomatic patients in unwittingly spreading the disease (thus causing community spread), and the fact that SARS-CoV-2 was much more than a respiratory affliction—it also affected the kidneys, the heart, the liver, and the brain.

The combined efforts of the world's scientific community resulted in the development of effective vaccines against Covid in an unprecedentedly short time—a little over a year. And not just one vaccine, but two dozen of them, most of which would remain effective as the coronavirus mutated. Throughout the pandemic, the science was solid; it was politics and corporate praxis that slowed down the availability of vaccines. As Jan-Werner Müller, a Princeton professor of political history and philosophy, lamented in the *London Review of Books* in April 2021, "no politician simply follows the science."

Variants / *New strains of the SARS-COV-2 coronavirus created by mutations within the virus's genome. Each new variant reacts differently with human cells, some dangerously enough to make the vaccines less effective than with previous versions.*

The first case of Covid-19 detected in the United States was caused by a variant. On January 21, 2020, a thirty-five-year-old man in Snohomish County, Washington, who had just returned from visiting Wuhan, China, came down with Covid-19. Analysis showed that he was infected with a variant of the original coronavirus—now called the ancestral strain—that had been identified a month earlier in Wuhan; the variant, called USA-WA1/2020, was similar to a version detected in other parts of China, specifically in the provinces of Fujian, Zhejiang, and Guangdong. The Wuhan ancestral strain had mutated and spread halfway around the world in less than a month, a foretaste of the enormity of the variant problem that would face epidemiologists in coming years.

That first US case did not, however, cause the spread of coronavirus in that country. Contact tracing showed that no one who had been in contact with the Snohomish County patient subsequently contracted Covid. According to Nicholas Christakis, in his book about the pandemic, *Apollo's Arrow*, "it seems that some other unknown person, possibly an American citizen with ties to China, arrived from Hubei Province around February 13 and seeded the outbreak in Washington with a different variant of the virus." It was this second carrier who became patient zero.

Almost every fresh outbreak of Covid-19 could be the result of a different variant, but five variants are known to have caused the most havoc so far. B.1.1.7 first mutated in Kent, England, in September 2020. Originally named VUI-202012/01, which meant "Virus Under Investigation in December 2020," and later renamed the "Alpha" variant (the WHO began naming variants after the Greek alphabet in May 2021), it probably formed in an immunocompromised patient who had had Covid-19 for several months; the longer a virus remains active in a human host, the more time it has to form multiple mutations, which is one of the reasons long Covid is such a concern (see "Long-Hauler").

The Alpha variant developed when the original coronavirus formed twenty-three mutations at more or less the same time (a phenomenon previously unknown to immunology—normally a virus forms one or two mutations a month). Eight of those mutations occurred in parts of the virus's genome that increased the virus's ability to bind with a human cell, making the variant more transmissible than the ancestral virus. The original coronavirus transmitted to about 10 percent of those who came into close contact with an infected person; B.1.1.7 transmitted to about 15 percent. Two of the mutations responsible for this increase were N501Y, which increased the firmness with which the virus's spike protein bonded to a human cell, and 69-70del, a mutation found in other viruses that could elude the human body's immune responses.

Three months after its appearance in southern England, the Alpha variant accounted for 75 percent of all new Covid-19 cases in the UK and had spread to thirty other countries, where it produced huge spikes of new cases, hospitalizations, and deaths. By May 2021, Alpha was similarly responsible for three-quarters of all new cases in the US.

Vaccines developed to treat the original coronavirus appeared to be less effective against the Alpha variant. Virologists determined, moreover, that unlike the original ancestral strain, the new variant was as virulent in young children as it was in teenagers and adults. A study conducted at the Schneider Children's Medical Center of Israel found that Alpha spread faster and more efficiently among children under nine than it did in adults. After Israel initiated its immunization program in December 2020, in which 57 percent of adults were immunized, new Covid cases continued to rise, although hospitalizations declined. The new cases were almost all among children infected with the Alpha variant.

A study published in the *British Medical Journal* *(BMJ)* in March 2021 found that "in addition to being more transmissible, [the Alpha variant] seems to be more lethal." The mortality rate for the original virus was 2.5 deaths per thousand cases; for the Alpha variant, it was 4.1.

Two other variants caused concern among health researchers. One, from South Africa, was named B.1.351, then renamed the "Beta" variant—and the other, from Brazil, was called B.1.1.28.1, or P.1 for short, and later the "Gamma" variant. Although Beta quickly became dominant in South Africa, the rate of infections in that country plummeted: new cases in the second week of March 2021 were about 1,200 a day, down from over 21,000 in January. The reasons were unknown, especially since a study published in *Nature* on March 8, 2021, reported that Beta was "markedly more resistant" to all vaccines than the ancestral coronavirus had been. Speculation had it that the country was closing in on herd immunity and that a nationwide lockdown in December and January had kept the infection rate down.

Comparing the situation in Brazil with that of South Africa underscored the need for strict restrictions. In March 2021, while new cases were plunging in South Africa, Brazil experienced a second wave that devastated the country. Even so, Brazilians continued to defy mask mandates and travel bans, following the example of their president, Jair Bolsonaro (nicknamed the "Tropical Trump"), who mocked those who advocated masks and told people concerned about the rising rate of infection to "stop being sissies." Mortality in Brazil achieved record highs in March, reaching 3,869 deaths a day, for a total of over 322,000 by the end of the month. The Gamma variant, detected in the northern city of Manaus in early 2021, was 2.2 times as transmissible as the original virus and could infect people who had already had Covid-19. That, combined with a painfully slow vaccine rollout, made the pandemic in Brazil an increasingly lethal reality.

The Delta variant, B.1.617.2, appeared in the western India state of Maharashtra in late 2020, and by February 2021 was linked to a staggering rise in the number of cases in that country—as many as 400,000 reported cases a day. It was a "double mutation," meaning that a single particle of the virus displayed mutations in two key areas of the spike protein. This made it more transmissible, according to virologist Shahid Jameel, who told the BBC on March 25 that a double mutation "may increase... risks and allow the virus to escape the immune system." This led doctors to suspect that the variant could infect persons who had been vaccinated and reinfect patients who had already contracted and recovered from Covid-19, a suspicion that turned out to be well-founded.

On April 26, Global News reported that thirty-six cases of Delta had been detected in Ontario, all of them associated with international travel, and by June the variant was found in every Canadian province and territory except Nova Scotia—even in Nunavut, where, in May, it was thought to be responsible for an outbreak at the Baffinland iron mine in Mary River Mine. Health authorities warned that it could become the dominant strain and possibly cause a fourth wave of the pandemic. A Queen's University mathematics professor predicted that by the end of July 2021, Delta would be responsible for 80 percent of cases in Ontario, and he proved to be right. On August 24, Ontario's new provincial health officer, Dr. Kieran Moore, announced that the Delta variant had become the dominant virus in the province and at least 90 percent of the population needed to be vaccinated if there were to be any chance of achieving herd immunity. On May 10, the WHO designated the Delta variant the fourth "variant of concern" when daily cases in England rose from 520 to 1,313 in one week. Subsequently, cases of the Delta variant showed up in seventy-four countries and on every continent but Antarctica.

In December 2020, a new variant was discovered in Nigeria and the UK. Named B.1.525, it contained two unique amino acid mutations in the spike protein that made it more resistant than other variants to vaccines. Writing in *Forbes,* former Harvard Medical School professor William A. Haseltine said that the new variant "deepens our uncertainty regarding the pandemic's future and our ability to control Covid-19." Within weeks, B.1.525 accounted for 20 percent of Nigeria's cases and had spread to thirteen other African countries, as well as the UK, France, and Canada.

Other "variants of interest," a designation less worrisome than "variant of concern," identified by the WHO include the Lambda variant (C.37), which first appeared in Peru in August 2020, and the Mu variant (B.1.621), which in August 2021 accounted for 39 percent of the active cases in Colombia and 13 percent of cases in Ecuador—and had shown up in Europe.

The fifth official variant of concern, B.1.1.529, was first reported in South Africa on November 24, 2021. It was the thirteenth variant overall but was named Omicron, after the fifteenth letter in the Greek alphabet. (The WHO skipped the letters Nu and Xi because Nu sounds like "new" and Xi is also a common family name in China.) Omicron exhibits thirty-six mutations on the spike protein, which make it much more transmissible than any of the previous variants. Two days after Omicron was detected in South Africa, that country had 2,465 new cases, and the variant had spread to seven other African countries.

Oddly, and perhaps ominously, on December 1, South Africa canceled its order of vaccines from Johnson & Johnson and from Pfizer, saying it had 16 million doses in storage, which was more than it could use. "There is a fair amount of apathy and hesitancy" in

Africa, Dr. Shabir Madhi, a South African vaccination expert, told the *New York Times*. Suspicion stemmed from decades of exploitation and poverty. That day, the *Times* also reported that Omicron accounted for 74 percent of all virus genomes sequenced in South Africa in November, and that Omicron had "overtaken Delta as the most prevalent variant" in the country.

Japan closed its borders to all foreigners on November 28, and the first cases showed up in Canada the next day. In the US, the first case of Omicron appeared in California in a man who'd been in South Africa on November 22. By then, there were 250,000 cases of Omicron worldwide. That turned out to be the tip of a very large iceberg: by mid-January 2022, the US alone was recording 800,000 new cases of Covid a day, and Omicron had overtaken Delta as the predominant Covid variant in the world, accounting for 99 percent of cases worldwide. On January 11, the WHO's regional director for Europe, Dr. Hans Kluge, called Omicron "a new west-to-east tidal wave."

In the early days, Omicron was thought to cause milder cases of Covid than Delta and to result in fewer hospitalizations and deaths. "For quite a while now," wrote American conservative journalist Jonah Goldberg in *The Dispatch* on December 3, "the hope for the long-term has been for the virus to evolve into something relatively harmless, like the cold, or at least relatively manageable, like the flu. As of now, Omicron looks a lot like that."

But the fond hopes of Republican anti-vaxxers that Omicron would be a sign that they'd been right to hold off was not to be realized. A study conducted by the Imperial College London (ICL) Covid-19 response team in December 2021, which included more than 300,000 cases in the UK, concluded not only that Omicron was more transmissible than Delta ("protection against reinfection by Omicron afforded by past infection may be as low as 19 percent"), but also that it was at least as severe. "The study finds no evidence of Omicron having lower severity than Delta," reported the ICL's news website, "judged by either the proportion of people testing positive who report symptoms, or by the proportion of cases seeking hospital care after infection."

As it turns out, Omicron is not a single variant but rather a "family" of subvariants. In January 2022, three subvariants had been identified—BA.1, BA.2, and BA.3—all three of which were first identified in South Africa. BA.1 has more than twenty extra mutations on its spike protein, allowing it to evade the defensive antibodies our immune system sends to attack it. In March 2022, as the wave caused by BA.1 began to recede, BA.2 began to spread in its wake. BA.2, with twenty-seven extra mutations, is known as a "stealth variant," because its genetic signature is the same as that of the Delta variant—PCR (polymerase chain reaction) tests cannot distinguish BA.2 from Delta. By the end of March, the BA.2 strain was dominant in Denmark, Nepal, and the Philippines, and was a major force in India, the UK, and South Africa. Altogether, it was accounting for 12 percent of new cases worldwide.

Studies of BA.2 suggest that a person who has had BA.1 is protected against contracting BA.2, and that two Pfizer and Moderna vaccinations are 70 percent effective against both BA.1 and BA.2. A booster shot provides 90 percent protection. Soaring cases of Covid in Hong Kong caused by BA.2 were not solely the result of the strain's high rate of transmission but also the result of vaccine hesitancy: 40 percent of Hong Kong residents were not vaccinated, and the death rate in March 2022—25 per 100,000 citizens—was the highest in the world.

In January and February 2022, two new members of the Omicron family, BA.4 and BA.5, were detected, again in South Africa. Both subvariants are usually discussed together, because the mutations in the spike proteins are identical. In March, the WHO placed both subvariants on its monitoring list. By April, BA.4 accounted for 35 percent of new cases in South Africa, and BA.5 accounted for 20 percent. The strains were also found in Austria, the UK, the US, Denmark, and Portugal. Though highly transmissible, they are thought to cause milder cases of Covid than their older siblings.

Plague / *Literally, a word referring to the contagion that swept through Europe periodically from the sixth to the seventeenth centuries. Figuratively, it is used to describe any affliction that causes suffering and damage. Also known as "the pox" and "the pest," from the French* la peste, *meaning the plague.*

On May 3, 2020, when the US death toll was 71,001, Donald Trump tweeted a strangely biblical-sounding prophecy: "And then came a Plague, a great and powerful Plague, and the World was never to be the same again! But America rose from this death and destruction, always remembering its many lost souls, and the lost souls all over the World, and became greater than ever before!"

Covid-19 is not the plague. The Black Death (as the plague was called) that devastated Europe in the Middle Ages—killing an estimated 25 million people in four years, at a time when the population of Europe was little more than 70 million—was caused not by a virus but by a bacterium, *Yersinia pestis*. A bacterium is a self-supporting, single-celled organism that can eat, grow, and reproduce on its own, whereas a virus is simply a set of genetic instructions coated in protein and wrapped in a liquid membrane that requires a living host in order to reproduce. A virus can only function by merging its genetic material with that of its host.

Plague caused by *Y. pestis* can take three forms: bubonic, when it invades the lymphatic system and

forms pustules, or buboes, in lymph nodes in the arm-
pits and groin; pneumonic, when it affects the lungs
(and when untreated is nearly always fatal); and septi-
cemic, when it enters the bloodstream. Bubonic plague
spills over to humans from rats—to some extent, but
not always, via fleas. The pneumonic form, however,
like a virus, can also be transmitted from human to
human by airborne droplets, direct physical contact,
or contaminated food or water. Studies have found that
75 percent of transmission during outbreaks of the
plague was human-to-human. Plague epidemics still
occur, usually in its bubonic form, in the Democratic
Republic of the Congo, Madagascar, Mongolia, and
Peru, accounting for about one hundred deaths per year.

Since the horrific days of the Black Death have
receded from our collective memory, we have taken
to referring to any catastrophe as a plague. But when
Moses called down the ten "plagues" of Egypt to
induce the Pharaoh to let his people go, not all of them
were contagious diseases. There were, for example, a
plague of frogs and a plague of red water (that was not
the Red Sea). Referring to them as plagues bumped
up the intensity of the situation. When Shakespeare's
Mercutio, in *Romeo and Juliet*, curses both the Cap-
ulets and the Montagues with "A plague o' both your
houses," we know that he is deeply injured.

At first, plagues were seen as inducements to being
good but soon switched to being punishments for
behaving badly. In Revelation 16, seven angels pour out

the "vials of the wrath of God," whereupon "men were scorched with great heat, and blasphemed the name of God, which hath power over these plagues." The plague that spread through London in 1665, as described by Daniel Defoe in *A Journal of the Plague Year*, was taken to be divine punishment inflicted on a sinful, or simply perplexed, population; in the days before the plague struck, writes Defoe, Londoners felt "it was a time of God's Anger, and dreadful Judgments were approaching; and that Despisers... should *wonder and perish*."

The present pandemic has likewise been interpreted in some circles as divine retribution. In March 2020, Patriarch Filaret, head of the Ukrainian Orthodox Church in Kyiv, told a Ukrainian television channel that the coronavirus was "God's punishment for the sins of men, the sinfulness of humanity." He went on to explain: "First of all, I mean same-sex marriage." The ninety-one-year-old patriarch tested positive for Covid-19 in September 2020, but recovered.

Vulnerable Populations / *People especially susceptible to infection because of such factors as age, health, living conditions, and other socioeconomic factors.*

Fourteen years before Covid-19, the *American Journal of Managed Care* noted that Americans living in poverty were much more likely to be in poor health and have disabling conditions than people living in more

affluent parts of the country. Other vulnerable populations included "the economically disadvantaged, racial
and ethnic minorities, the uninsured, low-income
children, the elderly, the homeless, those with human
immunodeficiency virus (HIV), and those with other
chronic health conditions, including severe mental illness... [and] rural residents." The article went on to
say that vulnerability to disease was "enhanced by race,
ethnicity, age, sex, and factors such as income, insurance coverage (or lack thereof), and absence of a usual
source of care," and included "those with chronic mental conditions, such as schizophrenia, bipolar disorder,
major depression, and attention-deficit/hyperactivity
disorder, as well as those with a history of alcohol and/
or substance abuse and those who are suicidal or prone
to homelessness... Overall, nonwhite women 45 to 64
years of age who are unemployed and uninsured with
lower incomes and education levels tend to report the
poorest health status."

The *Canadian Medical Association Journal* (*CMAJ*)
includes prisoners and refugees in this category, as
well as "those who are at risk of interpersonal violence,
and the Aboriginal communities that experience
shocking health inequalities." This means women in
abusive domestic relationships and residents of remote
Indigenous communities where health facilities are
inadequate or nonexistent.

When all these factors are added together, it's clear
that a large segment of Western society comprises

people who are highly susceptible to contagion from a rapidly proliferating, highly transmissible disease such as Covid-19. The phrase "accident waiting to happen" comes to mind, except that the situation is no accident. It's built into our society. It's collateral damage.

"Ideas about vulnerability shape the ways in which we manage and classify people, justify state intervention in citizens' lives, allocate resources in society and define our social obligations," Kate Brown writes in the journal *Ethics and Social Welfare* (2011). She goes on to say that " 'vulnerability' is so loaded with political, moral and practical implications that it is potentially damaging to the pursuit of social justice." The *CMAJ* warned that the concept of vulnerability "can be paternalistic and oppressive; it can serve to widen social control; and labelling groups as vulnerable can result in exclusion and stigmatization."

In other words, for groups that are vulnerable and may already feel excluded and stigmatized, the pandemic has served to draw our attention to their vulnerability. In the US, Black and Hispanic communities have been more affected by the pandemic than any other identifiable group, partly because people in those communities have limited access to health care and therefore tend to suffer from underlying health issues. (Other factors include the conviction on the part of some marginalized communities that anything coming from the government couldn't possibly be for their benefit.)

Princeton professor Keeanga-Yamahtta Taylor, writing in the *New York Times* (May 29, 2020) after the murder of George Floyd in Minneapolis four days earlier, notes that long-term vulnerability contributed to the fervor with which Black Americans rose in protest against police violence. "The coronavirus has scythed its way through Black communities," she writes, "highlighting and accelerating the ingrained social inequities that have made African-Americans the most vulnerable to the disease." By that time, APM Research Lab reported, Covid-19 had taken the life of one out of every 2,000 African-Americans—"a chilling affirmation," writes Taylor, "that Black lives still do not matter in the United States."

An unforeseen consequence of our conflicting notions of vulnerability arose during the debate about the projected order of vaccine recipients, when vaccines were developed. Most authorities agreed that the first to receive the vaccine, after the elderly and the immunocompromised, should be medical workers and national security personnel. But who would be next in line? Teachers? Pregnant women? Suggestions that the vaccine should go to vulnerable communities, most of whom were Black, Hispanic, or Indigenous, were met with resistance from white health professionals.

When vaccines eventually became available, the inequality of distribution became a pressing public issue. From the outset, it was clear that a higher percentage of white people were being vaccinated than either Black or Hispanic people in the US. By September 7, 2021, the Centers for Disease Control and Prevention (CDC) reported that nationwide, 56 percent of white people had received at least one dose of a vaccine, whereas only 48 percent of Hispanic people and 43 percent of Black people had. In some regions, the disparity was much greater. In Washington, D.C., for example, where Black people made up 71 percent of the deaths from Covid-19, they had received only 44 percent of the vaccinations.

Although by the end of 2021 many of these disparities had been addressed, the fact remains that the pandemic has underlined just how many citizens in North America's advanced society were, and remain, vulnerable.

Underlying Health Conditions / *Chronic health conditions that make infection with Covid-19 more dangerous than it would be in an otherwise healthy patient.*

"Underlying" means basic, or fundamental (think of rock formations). It is different from "preexisting," which is an insurance term for any health condition for which an applicant has received medical treatment before applying for an insurance policy—it was meant to preclude people who might actually need health insurance (such exclusions have been prohibited in the

US since the passage of the Affordable Care Act in 2010, but private insurance companies still apply them in Canada).

Underlying health conditions are diseases that put people who contract Covid-19 at greater risk of dying from it, and include such chronic diseases as diabetes, asthma, lung or liver disease, and cancer, as well as those that compromise the immune system, such as pneumonia, lupus, multiple sclerosis, or rheumatoid arthritis. Heart patients in Brazil who died after being administered hydroxychloroquine had underlying health conditions.

Studies indicate that people with obesity and Covid-19 are more likely to require hospitalization, to be admitted to intensive care, and to die than patients with a body mass index (BMI) under 30. Essentially, the higher a person's BMI, the greater the risk of severe reactions to Covid-19. According to Barry Popkin of the University of North Carolina, who in October 2020 conducted a meta-analysis of Covid risk, people with obesity "have more than double the likelihood of going into the hospital... and 50 percent more likelihood of dying." Obesity ranked with old age as a determining factor in the severity of Covid-19. People with obesity are also more likely to have other underlying health conditions, such as diabetes, lung disease, and hypertension, which makes them more susceptible to long-term damage from Covid-19. Studies also show that between 28 and 36 percent of the populations of the US, the UK, and Australia are obese. In Canada the figure is 26.8 percent and is climbing at the rate of 0.7 percent per year.

Although only 9 percent of the US population is asthmatic, people with asthma account for 11 percent of those testing positive for Covid-19. One reason for the overrepresentation might be that people with asthma tend to have themselves tested more often, because asthma symptoms are similar to those of Covid-19. But studies also show that of the two main types of asthma—allergic and non-allergic—it's the non-allergic asthma sufferers who have a significantly greater likelihood of contracting severe Covid-19. Gayatri Patel, of Northwestern University, who conducted one of the studies, thinks the answer might lie in the lungs' angiotensin-converting enzyme 2 (ACE2) receptors, the protein receptors that act as gateways through which coronaviruses enter human cells. There are more of them in the lungs of people with non-allergic asthma, and therefore more opportunities for the spike proteins on the coronavirus to attach to the cells.

Some patients with underlying health conditions have been advised to consult their physicians before receiving a Covid-19 vaccine. For example, people who are allergic to polyethylene glycol (PEG) may have a negative reaction to the Moderna and Pfizer vaccines, which contain that substance. However, the risk of anaphylactic shock from a reaction to PEG in a vaccine is almost infinitesimally small: according to Health Canada, of 1.8 million vaccine doses administered by the end of February 2021, only 50 (or about 0.0028 percent) produced anaphylactic reactions.

Pandemic /

> "Westchester matron and Bowery bum,
> Both shall dance with me when I rattle my drum."
> W. H. AUDEN, "Recitative by Death"

From the Greek pan *(all) and* demos *(the people), a pandemic is a multifocal infectious disease that has spread rampantly—originally throughout a region or a country, but now around the world. The World Health Organization declared Covid-19 a public health emergency of international concern on January 30, 2020, and a pandemic on March 11, 2020, a day when 7,059 new cases were reported worldwide.*

Pandemics are spread by travel; it may be that our innate fear and mistrust of strangers is the result of genetic memories of infectious diseases brought to our shores by travelers from abroad. The Greeks referred to all foreigners (*xénos*, as in xenophobia) as *barbarous*, or "barbarians," long before the plague arrived in Europe from Central Asia via caravans along the Silk Road or on ships arriving in trade ports in Italy and France. In the fourteenth century, the plague returned from Asia to kill up to half the population of

Europe; Italy and Normandy, both coastal regions, lost as many as 80 percent of their citizens in two years. As Frank M. Snowden remarks in *Epidemics and Society*, "shipping was essential to the spread of plague over long distances; this helps to explain the epidemiology of the disease—that is, its tendency to arrive in a country by ship and then to move inland by road and river traffic." In the twenty-first century, airplanes have replaced sailing ships, and people their cargo.

Plague epidemics persisted into the early 1900s. We don't hear about them so much in the Western world because they mainly affected poorer countries: India, China, and countries in Latin America. As Snowden relates, "the Centers for Disease Control and Prevention (CDC) reports that between 1900 and 2016, there were over one thousand cases of plague in the United States, concentrated in New Mexico, Arizona, Colorado, and California," carried mostly by hunters and campers who had come into contact with woodland rodents. And it was soldiers stationed at Camp Funston (now Fort Riley) in Kansas who spread the 1918 influenza pandemic to Europe and the rest of the world, when they were sent to the trenches in France.

Today, with people traveling more than ever, the Covid-19 pandemic is spread by way of international movement—through airports and on cruise ships, carried by tourists, business travelers, and migrant workers. As instanced by the reactions around the world, when a country goes into lockdown, the first things it locks down are its borders. New Zealand closed its borders to non–New Zealanders almost the day the world learned that the pandemic was afoot— China even before that.

A pandemic also crosses traditional borders between social and economic strata, emphasizing the disparity between rich and poor countries and citizens. The usual assumption is that the poor infect the rich, not the other way around. We say that the poor live in close quarters and have little access to health care, not that the rich hold large parties and indulge in international travel. But as Jamie Swift and Elaine Power note in *The Case for Basic Income*, the Covid-19 pandemic has created a " 'democratization' of insecurity," by which everyone, rich and poor, are equally vulnerable. Prime ministers, religious leaders, taxi drivers, and stock brokers have all been infected; the United States has been hit as hard as India. "The 2020 pandemic," they write, is both "a mirror and a spotlight, highlighting our society's brokenness."

David Quammen, the author of *Spillover,* an account of how animal diseases can be transmitted to humans, reminds us that placing the blame for this pandemic on others is an act of hypocrisy. We are all responsible for spreading animal-borne diseases. "What we eat," he told the *New York Times* in September 2020, "what we wear, all the other kinds of things that we buy... put varying degrees of pressure on the rest of the natural world." The more we chase after the world's resources—to make aluminum, or car tires, or cell phones—"the greater jeopardy we have of contacting all of the very diverse viruses that wild animals carry."

2

In These Uncertain Times

"Anxiety, stress, worry, fear, uncertainty,
dread, sadness, grief: these are all
normal and expected responses to a
massive disruptive event like a pandemic."

CANADIAN MENTAL HEALTH ASSOCIATION

Quarantine /

"There seems to be a plague upon the castle. All of us
are shriveling away. The butlers, the cooks, even our
little princess."

"The princess!" cried the plumber. "I must see her."

"No!" said the maid. "You must stay away from this
house. It is quarantined."

SHEILA HETI, "The Princess and the Plumber"

*To be accurate, it was the princess and her retainers who
were quarantined, not the house. A quarantine is the
removal of oneself or another from contact with others for
a specified period of time to avoid spreading a highly contagious disease.*

In medieval Latin, the name Quarantana was given to the mountain in the desert on which Jesus fasted alone for forty days and forty nights. The first recorded incidence of a government-mandated quarantine was in 1377, an early plague year in Europe (but not the first), when the port city of Ragusa (now Dubrovnik) decreed that crews on vessels arriving "from plague-infested areas shall not enter [Ragusa] or its district unless they spend a month on the islet of Mrkan or in the town of Cavtat, for the purpose of disinfection." A month wasn't forty days, but it was deemed close enough.

During the Covid-19 pandemic, quarantines were imposed in most countries in mid-March 2020, as travelers hastily returned to their countries of origin before the borders were closed. In Canada, returning travelers showing symptoms of Covid, and eventually all returnees, were strongly urged to self-isolate for fourteen days—a kind of mini-quarantine—under the federal Quarantine Act. Those returning to Canada and landing in Vancouver, Calgary, Toronto, or Montreal and connecting to their home destinations had to remain in isolation for fourteen days in a designated hotel in the city in which they landed before continuing their journeys.

On April 14, the government grew more insistent, saying that anyone entering Canada had to have "a credible quarantine plan" for self-isolation at home—a place where they could be isolated, with someone to bring them groceries, or whom they could call in an emergency—or else remain in a federally approved "quarantine location" for fourteen days before returning to their homes. By May 1, there were 330 travelers in quarantine locations, usually hotels, and hundreds more who were quarantined in disused military barracks in Trenton and Cornwall, Ontario, for the purpose of disinfection. In the US, "quarantine stations" were set up for arriving travelers in twenty ports of entry and land border crossings throughout the country, in which CDC officers assessed travelers' suitability to enter. Anyone deemed too sick to enter was placed in quarantine.

In the UK, mandatory quarantines for travelers from high-risk countries were introduced in February 2021. There were, at the time, thirty-three countries on the UK's high-risk list, most of them in South America or Africa, although Portugal was also on the list. In the Republic of Ireland, buses ferried passengers from airports to designated "quarantine hotels," escorted by members of the Irish Defence Forces. Each detainee was charged 1,875 euros for the twelve-night stay, or else had to pay a 2,000 euro fine for failure to comply. By the time the quarantine requirement was lifted, on September 25, 2021, more than 10,000 people had been quarantined.

Stringent though these measures were, they were better than the way the city of London enforced quarantines during plague years in previous centu-ries. In *1606*, historian James Shapiro recounts that houses in which a plague victim lived were sealed with everyone in the victim's family inside them, includ-ing servants, and the front doors were painted with a red X—at first with a water-based paint, but when that kept being washed off, the X was repainted with an oil-based paint. Guards watched to make sure no one tried to leave. Residents remained inside their houses until either the victims recovered or everyone died of starva-tion or, more often, the plague. Anyone caught outside a plague house was flogged; anyone with plague symp-toms caught outside the house was executed.

Passengers and crew members aboard the cruise ship *Diamond Princess* might have felt that the 1606 protocols were back in place. The ship was quarantined in the Port of Yokohama on February 3, 2020, when ten passengers tested positive for Covid-19 (the first major outbreak outside China). In all, 712 passengers and crew from a total of 3,711 people on board were infected, and fourteen of them died.

By March 1, everyone on board had been removed to hospitals in or around Tokyo, and they were eventually returned to their own countries, where they were again quarantined. American writer Gay Courter was one of those on board and later wrote a book about the ordeal entitled *Quarantine!* At first, she said in a CBC inter-view, "people seemed more upset about changing their travel plans than getting the virus." When the captain announced that ten people had tested positive and the ship was under quarantine—"a word I had thought was obsolete"—all passengers were confined to their cabin for fourteen days.

When the ship's quarantine was lifted, virologists were able to study virus samples taken from infected passengers and crew. They found that the original coronavirus had undergone a total of twenty-four mutations and that these new variations had infected 64.2 percent of those who contracted Covid-19. This was extremely swift evolution, giving the scientists a frightening portent of what this novel coronavirus was capable of when its hosts were in a tightly confined environment. In three weeks, it had branched off into five subgroups, each with a unique variant of the disease, and each potentially requiring a different epidemiological approach. Normally, the Covid coronavirus mutates more slowly than the seasonal flu—about twenty-five mutations per year, compared with the flu's fifty—but in enclosed places like a cruise ship, a prison, or a long-term care facility, mutations occur much more frequently. And that can potentially produce a new form of the coronavirus that is resistant to vaccines.

Long-Term Care Facility /

"The weight of this sad time we must obey...
The oldest hath borne most." *King Lear,* Act 5, Scene 3

"Long-term care facility" (LTCF) is an unintentionally ironic name for a multi-residence home for the aged; according to the National Care Planning Council, the average length of stay in a nursing home in the US is only 835 days. In Ontario, the wait list for long-term stay includes, on average, 35,308 names, and the usual wait time is only 152 days. In Europe, stays in LTCFs are also short; a study published in the British Medical Journal (BMJ) *in April 2020 found that the average length of residence in an LTCF in six European countries was 513.8 days and that 42 percent of those admitted to an LTCF in Europe died within the first year. And all that was before Covid.*

The first person to die of Covid-19 in Canada was an eighty-year-old man living in the Lynn Valley Care Centre in North Vancouver. He died on March 8, 2020, and two months later, 82 percent of the more than 3,000 people who had died from Covid-19 in Canada were residents of Canada's 2,039 long-term care facilities, even though LTCF residents accounted for only 1 percent of the total population.

In the fall of 2019, before anyone had even heard of Covid-19, the National Institute on Ageing issued a report stating that long-term care homes in Ontario were underfunded, overcrowded, and chronically understaffed. Part-time staff were working at several facilities and traveling back and forth between them to earn a decent wage, thereby increasing the risk of inter-facility contamination. A subsequent submission by the Ontario Long Term Care Association warned that the industry was at "a tipping point."

When the pandemic arrived in Canada, LTCF residents began dying in greater-than-average numbers, and health-care workers in such facilities were among the highest-risk groups in the country. In one private facility in Quebec, the Résidence Herron, patients who became ill between March 26 and April 16, 2020, were left unattended in their beds because the facility's staff had walked out: thirty-eight patients died. The situation across Canada worsened as the death toll rose rapidly everywhere, but especially in nursing homes in Ontario and Quebec. In May, the federal government assigned 1,300 Armed Forces personnel to assist—in reality, to replace—workers in twenty-seven facilities in Quebec and five in Ontario. The personnel reported gross irregularities in the facilities: poor practices for dealing with infection, neglect of residents, resentment and cruelty among staff, malnutrition in residents, even cockroaches. Newspapers began referring to the facilities as "houses of horror."

This situation ought not to have been a surprise. Two years earlier, Bethe Wettlaufer, a registered nurse working in a home in Woodstock, Ontario, had been found guilty of eight counts of first-degree murder and six counts of attempted murder: for nine years, she'd been deliberately killing her charges by injecting them with high doses of insulin. The inquiry into the case, headed by Honourable Justice Eileen Gillese, included ninety-one recommendations focusing on changes required to make the system work better. Most were ignored. As Kelly McParland, writing about the report in the *National Post* in August 2019, put it, "if you have a loved one in long-term care in Ontario, you better keep a close watch on them, because the system sure won't."

When the second wave of Covid-19 struck in September 2020, little had changed. According to York University sociologist Pat Armstrong, Canada's record was dismal because the majority of the country's LTCFs are privately owned and operated, resulting in "under-training and poor treatment of workers, substandard and ageing facilities, overcrowding, and poor infection control capabilities." In Ontario, 58 percent of LTCFs are privately owned, and two-thirds of those are run by for-profit companies.

By March 2021, deaths in LTCFs accounted for 69 percent of all deaths in Canada, compared with an average of 41 percent worldwide. And the crisis, like the pandemic itself, had spread beyond Ontario and Quebec; in a *Maclean's* article published in April, Stephen Maher reported that "Saskatchewan had only two resident deaths in the first wave, but 84 in the second. Manitoba had three, then 468. Alberta went from 153 deaths to 1,013. The province now leads Canada with the highest percentage of its homes experiencing outbreaks."

The situation elsewhere in the world was similar to that in Canada. In the US, although LTCFs accounted for only 4 percent of Covid cases overall, deaths in those facilities accounted for 31 percent of the national total. In Australia, long-term care residents accounted for 7.5 percent of all Covid cases but 75.3 percent of Covid deaths. In the UK, one of every twenty residents of LTCFs contracted Covid, and one in five of those died. By the end of October 2021, 22,948 more LTCF residents had died than in any of the previous five years.

The coronavirus pandemic proved that LTCFs were virtual incubation chambers awaiting infection. They were more reminiscent of nineteenth-century pesthouses, where diseased victims were sent to die, than of modern health institutions. The telling statistic, recorded by Stephen Maher in *Maclean's*, might be that many of those who died in LTCFs "died not of Covid-19 but from dehydration, starvation, injuries, or improper care." It is undoubtedly true that, as Dr. Samir K. Sinha, the National Institute on Ageing's director of health policy research, stated in December 2021, "Covid-19 devastated Canada's long-term care and retirement homes." But it is also true that it had a lot of help.

Personal Protective Equipment (PPE) / *Protective equipment worn by health-care professionals in hospitals and nursing homes. These prophylactic items include face masks and shields, gowns, respirators, gloves, and even full-body suits to prevent wearers from contracting or spreading Covid-19. Most of these items were also worn by the general public.*

Early in the pandemic, in the absence of vaccines, governments around the world urged citizens to wear personal protective equipment, especially face masks, and to exercise other safety measures, such as handwashing and social distancing, in the event of exposure to people who might be carrying the disease. Frontline workers—paramedics and the medical and support staff in hospitals, test clinics, nursing homes, and long-term care facilities—were the most vulnerable to infection and were strongly advised to use PPE at all times when on duty.

The problem was that many hospitals and nursing facilities did not have enough PPE to go around. In March 2020, the WHO announced that shortages of PPE were "endangering health workers worldwide." The WHO had shipped half a million PPE sets to forty-seven countries in Asia, the Middle East, and Africa but that was just a drop in the bucket: the organization estimated that the world needed 89 million medical masks per month, as well as 76 million gloves and

1.6 million goggles. It urged the manufacturers of protective equipment to increase production by 40 percent.

By the end of that month, shortages around the world had become critical. In Italy, sixty-one doctors died after contracting Covid-19 because of a lack of adequate PPE. In Spain, where PPE shortages were severe, at least 12,000 health-care professionals came down with the disease. The French government seized hundreds of thousands of face masks that had been hoarded by people hoping to resell them online. In India, doctors were protecting themselves with raincoats and swimming goggles. And in hospitals in the Philippines, gowns were in such short supply that hospital staff were wearing plastic garbage bags over their scrubs.

In the United States, when then-president Donald Trump finally acknowledged the pandemic's existence in April 2020, he blamed former president Barack Obama for failing to stockpile PPE in anticipation of a pandemic. It then emerged that Obama's administration had, in fact, left an adequate supply of PPE, and it was Trump's team that had emptied the cupboard. Back in January 2020, Lawrence Wright records in *The Plague Year*, the planes that were sent to China to evacuate Americans from Wuhan "were filled with eighteen tons of PPE, including masks, gowns, and gauze." In July, the lack of PPE in the United States became critical: nurses were washing masks and face protectors without knowing if they would still be effective. "It's almost five months into a pandemic," said Deborah Burger, copresident of National Nurses United, on July 9, the day the US reached a record 59,400 new cases, "in the richest country in the world, and we're putting people's lives at risk because we don't have enough PPE."

By that time, the law of supply and demand meant that the cost of PPE had risen dramatically. Medical face masks had gone up sixfold, N95 respirator masks had tripled, and the cost of hospital gowns had doubled. China was able to sell the same masks, gowns, and gauze that Trump had sent them back to the US at a tidy profit.

3M, one of the companies that manufactures N95 masks in the US, reported that its first quarter net sales in 2021 were up 9.6 percent—to $8.85 billion. Such staggering figures caused a surge of fake N95 masks and respirators. In February, US Customs seized 15 million counterfeit N95 masks coming into the States from China. In Ontario, when the government became aware of possible fake N95 masks in its provincial stockpile—some with counterfeit 3M stickers on the boxes—it suspended distribution to hospitals until the inventory had been checked and cleared. It's impossible to know how many people came down with Covid during the delay, but every day brought new cases and deaths.

Some businesses made their staff pay for their own PPE; others passed the cost of providing staff with PPE on to their customers. In February 2021, the *Washington Post* reported that dentists and hair salons in some states were adding five-dollar "disinfecting fees" to their customers' bills, and some long-term care facilities also made their staff supply their own PPE. In Michigan, the attorney general's office issued a cease and desist order to eleven long-term care facilities after forty-five residents complained that they'd been charged nine hundred dollars extra for "supplemental Covid-19 fees."

Whether because of incompetence or perfidy, PPE shortages have remained a global problem throughout the pandemic. In the US, the federal government regularly publishes a list of medical supply shortages for the information of both suppliers and purchasers; nine months into the pandemic, the list still included hospital ventilators as well as surgical gloves, gowns, and other apparel. The reason given in each case was "increased demand," a euphemism for "we had no idea we'd need so many." In response, companies that traditionally manufactured other items retooled their assembly plants to produce PPE. In Canada, for example, Bauer—the hockey equipment manufacturer—began making plastic face shields. Hewlett-Packard programmed 3D printers to print thousands more shields. Samuelsohn, a Montreal-based luxury clothing manufacturer, retooled its production lines to produce hospital gowns. And Irving Oil, the largest gasoline company in the Atlantic provinces, shifted some of its facilities to making hand sanitizer.

These were all catch-up maneuvers made necessary by a lack of preparedness for and a painfully slow reaction to the pandemic. To borrow a military metaphor, Covid-19 remained an invisible enemy far too long into the conflict. Frank M. Snowden, in *Epidemics and Society*, quotes microbiologist Joshua Lederberg: "In the contest between humans and microbes, the only defense humans possess is their wits." In a country like the US, whose chief strategy in wartime has been to seek and destroy, the pandemic's microbes were easily able to come in under the radar. When intelligence and diplomacy were needed, America had Donald Trump.

Face Mask / *A covering over the nose and mouth, like the surgical masks worn by hospital staff, to reduce the range of potentially virus-laden droplets in the wearer's breath.*

Originally, both American and Canadian health authorities said there was no need to wear face masks in public unless you had Covid-19, but since there was little testing at the time, no one knew if they had it. The concern was that a mass public run on personal protective equipment would deplete the supply available to medical professionals in hospitals and long-term care facilities, who were dealing with infected patients daily—which is exactly what happened anyway.

In early April 2020, when it became clear that Covid-19 was being transmitted by people who were asymptomatic—and, perhaps equally important, that surgical masks were in woefully short supply in hospitals and nursing homes—the US Centers for Disease Control and Prevention and Dr. Theresa Tam, Canada's chief public health officer, changed their messages: everyone should wear a face mask in public. Cloth masks, they said, were adequate. They even posted instructions on how to make them. Overnight, people were sewing masks for themselves and their families, and "how-to" YouTube videos proliferated. Face masks became ubiquitous, then fashionable, and then symbolic.

"The wearing of masks has become... politicized," *Forbes* reported on May 14, 2020. Evidence from the *Proceedings of the National Academy of Sciences* and *Nature* showed that wearing a face mask protected others from contact with one's own germs (not so much the other way around) and that therefore wearing a mask was mostly a mark of concern for others. Websites showed celebrities wearing face masks with messages on them: Arnold Schwarzenegger's said, "We'll Be Back" and Olivia Newton-John's said, "#Masking For A Friend." Donald Trump, at political rallies that his own office said he was not supposed to be holding, handed out face masks emblazoned with the campaign slogan "Keep America Great"—but only to attendees who'd made donations to his campaign fund.

Wearing a mask remained a political statement throughout the pandemic. Jonathan Weisman wrote in the *New York Times* on January 12, 2022, "If you're in the capital, and you see somebody without a mask on, you say, 'Oh—that's a Republican.' "

When an object becomes politicized, it takes on new meaning. During the anti–Vietnam War demonstrations in the 1960s and 1970s, those opposed to the US presence in Vietnam began wearing military clothing purchased at army surplus stores as a protest against those wearing uniforms because they were in the army. Having long hair and a fatigue jacket with jeans and a T-shirt was a sign that you were against the war. (I went so far as to wear a khaki army tie with my paisley shirts.)

Face masks are traditionally worn to disguise one's true identity: the Lone Ranger, Zorro, Batman and Robin, the Phantom of the Opera, and, more recently, Zapatistas in Mexico and members of the Antifa movement (short for *Antifaschistische Aktion*, or anti-fascist action, which Trump tried to have declared a terrorist organization) have all worn them for this reason. As the pandemic continued, however, wearing a face mask identified the wearer as someone who was following science-based, medical recommendations for slowing the spread of Covid-19, whereas not wearing one identified the person as someone who, for one reason or another, was ignoring those recommendations.

In June 2020, when the *New York Times* ran a front-page photograph of a Black woman at a lunch counter wearing a mask as she served coffee to a white man who was not wearing one, Adam Shatz, the US editor of the *London Review of Books*, remarked that he considered the photo "a reminder that Jim Crow hasn't so much died as been reconfigured."

Those who refused to wear face masks, however, were making an ambiguous statement. Some genuinely mistrusted the science, believing either that there was no pandemic or that masks didn't help. There were also left-wing anarchists who rejected all forms of government control. Right-wing, pro-Trump scofflaws considered measures to quell the pandemic a Democrat-led plot to undermine Trump's authority. All camps could be dangerously self-righteous. In Van Nuys, California, a Target employee was severely beaten by two customers who refused to wear face masks, and in Flint, Michigan, a dollar store employee was shot and killed because he insisted a customer wear a mask.

On March 2, 2021, the governors of Texas and Mississippi, both Republicans, announced that they were lifting their mandates on mask wearing and social distancing and allowing stores and restaurants to reopen at full capacity. President Biden, at a press conference the next day, said that lifting restrictions in Texas when the state was reporting 7,000 new cases a day was anti-science. "The last thing we need," said Biden, "is the Neanderthal thinking that, in the meantime, everything's fine, take off your mask." Some suggested that was an insult to Neanderthals.

Mississippi governor Tate Reeves replied that although he had officially lifted the mandate, the precautions hadn't changed, and he hoped people would continue to wear masks. All that had changed, he said, was that "the government is no longer telling you what you can and cannot do." The government, however, still told people to wear seat belts, to not drive faster than a specific speed, and to report their incomes for purposes of being taxed. Balking at wearing a face mask was illogical, more a matter of faith than reason, and refusing to mandate the practice had nothing to do with being a laissez-faire government.

Compared with the fluid realm of politics, the science behind face masks was solid. Studies showed that they did slow down the spread of Covid. The *Nature* study cited above found that, on average, fluid droplets from a contagious person contained 7 million viruses per milliliter, and a person emitted 2,600 such droplets per minute during a normal conversation, and much more when shouting—for example, at a Donald Trump rally. During the Beijing Winter Olympics in February 2022, at the height of the Omicron surge, spectators watching events from the grandstands were told by officials they could clap but not yell. Virus-laden droplets may hang in the air for up to eight minutes, and even longer in cold air. In winter, a person could come into contact with the virus just by walking through the same spot as someone with Covid-19, even up to an hour later. This makes measures such as contact tracing almost impossible; the highly contagious virus can be detected but, like a fingerprint, the evidence lingers after the culprit is long gone.

Wearing a mask during a pandemic sends two signals: you trust science, and you care about the health of others. Wearing a face mask, writes Megan Garber in *The Atlantic*, "is to engage in a basic but highly visible act of altruism." Not wearing one, or wearing one pulled down under your nose, could mean anything from "I'm invincible," to "I don't think anyone around me is infectious," to "I hate all forms of government and will make my own decisions," or "I love Donald Trump and don't give a damn about anyone else." All the reasons for not wearing a mask are flawed: no one is invincible, we can never know whether someone near us is infectious, not all government mandates threaten our human rights, and many avid Trump supporters contracted Covid-19 and died.

Do cloth masks work as well as other kinds? Most health experts are lukewarm about cloth masks, but not all non-cloth masks are equal. Dr. Christopher Labos, writing in the *Montreal Gazette* on April 7, 2020, noted that "there is precious little evidence that non-medical cloth masks prevent disease." He cited a

2013 test that found that surgical masks were three times as effective as cloth masks at blocking virus particles. Still, he wrote, wearing a cloth mask was "better than nothing." A more recent study, conducted in Bangladesh, found that wearing a surgical mask decreased one's chance of contracting Covid by 11.2 percent, whereas wearing a cloth mask decreased it by 5 percent.

According to the CDC, N95 or KN95 masks, made from electrostatic polypropylene fiber, are the most effective: both offer up to 95 percent protection from either large or small particles. A CDC study conducted in California over a nine-month period in 2021, and published in February 2022, found that people wearing N95 and KN95 masks were 83 percent less likely to test positive for Covid, and that the difference between wearing a cloth mask and not wearing any mask at all was "not statistically significant."

The only difference between N95 and KN95 masks is that N95 masks are approved in the US by the National Institute for Occupational Safety and Health (NIOSH), whereas the KN95 masks are approved by the Food and Drug Administration, or FDA. Surgical masks, also cleared by the FDA, are better than cloth masks, which are neither tested nor regulated and can be made of many different types of cloth. Not all cloth types have the same level of filtration. Unless you have an N95 or a KN95 mask, the best protection is from double masking with surgical masks. If you want to make a fashion statement other than "I trust science and I care about other people," you can wear a cloth mask printed with a motto of your choice over an N95 or KN95 mask.

Alma Möller, Iceland's director of health, told Elizabeth Kolbert of the *New Yorker* in June 2020 that masks are less effective than a good tracking system. Möller believed that wearing a mask might be advisable for someone who is actively showing symptoms, but that such persons shouldn't be outside anyway. "We think [masks] don't add much," she said, "and they can give a false sense of security." Iceland thought its highly efficient tracking system and small population would work in the country's favor, and for a while it appeared so: by February 2021, Iceland had had only twenty-nine deaths, even though it had not gone into lockdown and had not closed its borders to tourists. But in the early summer of 2021—Covid-19's third wave—restrictions including the wearing of masks in public were imposed. They were lifted on June 26, when 71 percent of the population was at least partially vaccinated, but were reimposed on July 24, as a small surge of Covid-19 cases swept the country. As the world learned during the Omicron surge, tracking systems can be quickly overwhelmed; face masks are forever.

Few countries were able to imitate Iceland's efficient tracking system anyway, and even in those that could— New Zealand, for example—wearing face masks was mandated. In New Zealand, a government publication issued in February 2021 stipulated that everyone over the age of twelve "legally must wear a face covering: on public transport; on domestic flights; by taxi and ride-share drivers." By July, New Zealand had one of the world's best records for Covid: 2,742 cases and only twenty-six deaths in a population of 5 million. By then, most countries had mandated face masks and social distancing (although with the proviso "as much as possible" to allow some wiggle room for the disinclined) on public transport and in other government-controlled venues. It was this wiggle room—"we strongly advise"; "health authorities recommend"; "when possible"—that took the urgency out of the rules and made governments appear to be waffling on issues of public safety.

Handwashing / *Another of the recommended means of slowing the spread of Covid-19, along with mask wearing and social distancing.*

Early in the pandemic, before much was known about the means by which Covid-19 spread so quickly, health authorities urged frequent handwashing because they believed the virus could live on surfaces such as door handles, stair rails, and tabletops (contaminated surfaces are known in medical circles as "fomites"), as bacteria and some other viruses can. Norovirus—a highly infectious virus that kills more than 200,000 people a year—is spread by touching fomites and then the mouth (it is most dangerous among children under five), and respiratory syncytial virus (RSV), which causes wheezing pneumonia in children, is spread by both particle droplets and contaminated surfaces. The virus responsible for avian flu has been detected on stainless steel surfaces up to 144 hours after contact, and in humid conditions, bacteria such as *Staphylococcus* and *Streptococcus* can linger on dry surfaces for several months. So it made sense for researchers to urge people to frequently wash their hands and wipe down solid objects.

Subsequent studies, however, showed that the novel coronavirus is spread almost entirely by aerosol particles. People didn't wash as many milk cartons and doorknobs after that, but handwashing was still recommended; in January 2021, when Public Health England updated its guidelines for slowing the spread of Covid-19, it placed handwashing at the top of its list. As *The Guardian* noted, handwashing doesn't hurt, and it prevents a number of other infectious diseases, including many hospital-acquired infections. Because of overcrowding and international travel, the importance of hand hygiene has increased in recent decades and is reflected in the medical literature. The number of publications promoting hand sanitizing increased from 4 per year in the 1950s to 554 per year in the early 2010s. The CDC website advises that "handwashing is one of the best ways to protect yourself and your family from getting sick."

Although most countries encouraged frequent handwashing, in many poorer nations, regular hand hygiene was almost impossible. According to data compiled by the World Bank, 97.4 percent of Iraqis had access to facilities with soap and water, for example, but only 8.2 percent of Ethiopians did, as well as 1.2 percent of Liberians and 4.6 percent of Rwandans. In such countries, face masks and social distancing remain the principal defenses against contagion.

Early in the pandemic, I took to carrying a small bottle of hand sanitizer when I went out. Most stores still put large containers of it at their entrances, accompanied by signs saying, "Please use." The sites are unmonitored, and no one knows how effective these measures have been, but most people use them without demur. Before Covid-19, alcohol-based hand rub was favored over soap and water, but now these commercial hand sanitizers have been deemed insufficient. "Alcohol-based hand sanitizers can quickly reduce the number of microbes on hands in some situations," advises the CDC, "but sanitizers do *not* eliminate all types of germs." A 2019 study found that hand sanitizer's ability to inactivate the influenza A virus was significantly reduced when mucus (sputum) was present; influenza A remained active in sputum after two minutes of sanitizer use. I've never seen anyone apply hand sanitizer at an entrance to a retail store for two minutes.

Ordinary soap, however, is a natural virucide. As Brooke Jarvis writes in the *New Yorker* (August 3 and 10, 2020), "the hydrophobic tails of soap molecules bond with the lipid membrane that protects the virus, literally ripping it apart, while their hydrophilic heads bond with the water that washes the dead virus away." Covering your hands with soap suds—for as long as it takes to remember whether the last instructions you read said fifteen seconds or twenty seconds—should do the trick.

In January 2020, before the pandemic reached the United States, the US Food and Drug Administration (FDA) sent a warning letter to Gojo Industries about its claims that its product, Purell hand sanitizer, was effective against viruses such as Ebola, norovirus, and influenza. "The FDA is currently not aware of any adequate and well-controlled studies demonstrating that killing or decreasing the number of bacteria or viruses on the skin by a certain magnitude produces a corresponding clinical reduction in infection or disease caused by such bacteria or virus." In other words, even if the hand sanitizer reduced the amount of virus on a person's hands, it still didn't mean that that person wouldn't contract the disease caused by that virus, because the virus is mostly airborne. Gojo removed the claim from its Purell labels.

A study conducted in the US in April 2020 by Bradley Corporation—a company that sells commercial hygiene equipment—found that 90 percent of respondents said they closely followed CDC recommendations to wash their hands and 78 percent said they were washing their hands at least six times a day. Most people said they would continue hand hygiene after the pandemic ended. Some of those who commented on the study found these results "suspicious."

Social Distancing / *Maintaining a distance of six feet (or two meters) from other people; or one meter in most Asian countries; or a meter and a half in Mexico; or "the length of one alligator" in Leon County, Florida; or four ravens in the Canadian North; or three raccoons in Toronto; or the wingspan of a bald eagle on the University of British Columbia campus. Government-mandated social distancing measures also included school and workplace closures, cancellation of public events, and stay-at-home orders.*

In early March 2020, the CDC in the US recommended "limiting face-to-face contact with others." Health Canada followed suit at the same time that restrictions were imposed on social gatherings. Provincial and state governments closed shopping malls, restaurants, theaters, and concert halls. When those amenities partially reopened in May 2020, many health advisers warned people to continue social distancing.

Most governments and health officials pulled back from issuing outright marching orders, preferring to present restrictions as recommendations rather than as mandates. In the US, the Johns Hopkins advisory for Covid-19, dated July 15, 2020, defined "social distancing" as "staying home and away from others as much as possible." The Covid-19 website of the Australian Capital Territory (ACT) government is similarly cautious in its wording: "Physical distancing means separating yourself from others as much as possible." In the UK, even those who were self-isolating after exposure to Covid during the Omicron surge were simply advised that if they *had* to leave their homes, they *"should* maintain social distancing... and wear a face covering *where possible*" (my italics). Except in China and Australia, this was the tone throughout most of the pandemic.

It was kind of quaint, the notion that left to our own devices, most of us would do the right thing. It's a faint echo of the idea behind the economic philosophy of the eighteenth-century Scottish economist Adam Smith, whose *The Wealth of Nations* held that by eliminating restrictions to trade and pricing, governments would ultimately advance the cause of the common good. When everyone acted in their own self-interest, Smith believed, the general well-being of society as a whole would be achieved. The appearance of Smith's book in 1776 coincided with the American Revolution, and

Americans grabbed the ideas of minimal government interference and the sanctity of self-interest and ran with them.

Unfortunately, the ideas didn't work in the field of economics—the world has more trade and pricing restrictions now than ever before in history—and their application to social situations hasn't worked either. As we learned during the Trump years, without specific restrictions, it takes only a minority of people doing the wrong thing to nullify efforts by the majority to do the right thing. In a pandemic, the refusal of a small percentage of the population to wear masks, maintain social distance, or be vaccinated ensures that the infection will spread at its wonted pace among the population as a whole.

For example, a study published in the journal *PLOS ONE* found a direct correlation between the imposition of social distancing polices in twenty-seven European countries and subsequent declines in new Covid cases. Social distancing policies reduced population mobility, and that resulted in fewer new cases. A 10 percent decrease in mobility—fewer people going out to stores, restaurants, concerts, and so on—was followed by an 11.8 percent decrease in new Covid cases two weeks later; a 50 percent decrease in mobility led to a 46.6 percent decrease in new cases two weeks later. Social distancing policies work, the study concluded; the authors also added that mandated policies work better than non-mandated policies.

Most retail outlets that reopened in May 2020 followed social distancing guidelines by limiting the number of customers allowed on the premises, that number depending on the size of the outlet (sometimes it was just one), and by painting footprints on the floor at checkout counters that were six feet apart, to suggest to customers where they should stand. Government and hospital waiting areas, airport departure lounges, and theaters taped off seats so that passengers and patients could maintain at least a semblance of social distancing. Most restaurants reduced their number of tables and found creative ways to allow enough customers in to make staying open profitable. Many, such as Amsterdam's Mediamatic ETEN, constructed a mini-greenhouse around each outdoor table so that customers could avoid close encounters with other tables—with the added benefit of being able to dine during rainstorms. The Inn at Little Washington, a restaurant in Virginia, placed interestingly dressed mannequins at tables throughout the dining area so that socially distanced customers wouldn't feel lonely. "I've always had a thing for mannequins," owner Patrick O'Connell told a local news station. "You can have lots of fun dressing them up, and they never complain about anything."

Even so, just as many people resisted face mask mandates, many also resisted social distancing regulations. Because, in its first wave, Covid-19 swept mainly through elderly populations and low-income communities where proper social distancing was next to impossible, young people from higher-income areas tended to feel the regulations didn't apply to them.

Social distancing mandates disproportionately hurt bars and restaurants. To an industry always hovering on the edge of bankruptcy, the pandemic threatened to deliver the coup de grâce to a large number of establishments. By the end of 2020, more than 110,000 restaurants had closed in the US, and 10,000 folded in Canada. According to the National Restaurant Association in the US, another 500,000 were on the brink of closing permanently; the industry, said the association, was "in an economic freefall."

When governments did mandate social distancing restrictions and daily inspections, many restaurant owners and their customers found ways to survive. But their survival also helped enable the pandemic to stay alive. Customers wore masks while entering and leaving the restaurant but not while sitting at their tables—which was most of the time. Outside, customers dined in huts and tents and yurts and glass houses, enclosures in which people sat in close contact, unmasked, and often without adequate ventilation. Covid-19 continued to spread.

Covid also spread when social distancing restrictions were lifted. On March 5, 2021, a year into the pandemic, the *New York Times* reported the results of research conducted by the CDC. "Federal researchers also found that [US] counties opening restaurants for on-premises dining—indoors or outdoors—saw a rise in daily infections about six weeks later, and an increase in Covid-19 death rates about two months later."

But self-interest often trumps good sense. In a *New Yorker* article on March 1, 2021, staff writer Nick Paumgarten admits that "it may be, during this Covid year, that no one should be dining at restaurants at all, outside or inside," but also notes that many people, including him, did. Paumgarten describes his experience in October 2020, when dining at a New York restaurant called Hamido: "The evening was mild, and the curve was still more or less flat; happy to be around people other than our families, we sat at a large table on the sidewalk, in the open air, sharing platters of bran-grilled orate, grilled octopus, fried sardines, baba ghanoush, and beers of our own bringing. Was all this reckless? Probably. But we are nothing if not weak."

That month, in New York City, the number of deaths from Covid-19 had flattened to an average of thirteen a day. But by mid-December, the daily toll had again risen to over one hundred.

Whether or not social distancing restrictions were enforced depended on where and who you were. Between March 17 and May 4, 2020, the New York police arrested forty people for social distancing violations, from sitting on porches to attending memorial services. Of those, thirty-five were Black, four were Hispanic, and one was white.

Community Spread / *When people become infected with the virus without having had known contact with an infected person; the point at which the pandemic's spread becomes untraceable, and therefore uncontrollable.*

On March 24, 2020, Dr. Theresa Tam, Canada's chief public health officer, announced that 53 percent of the country's cases were the result of community spread, a realization, she said, that called for "a fundamental shift in our epidemiology." Until then, it was believed that by tracking infection routes from infected to uninfected persons and then finding, testing, and isolating those potentially contagious persons, epidemiologists could control the spread.

That strategy doesn't work when health authorities don't know who in the community is passing on the disease. A week after Dr. Tam's announcement, community spread accounted for up to 65 percent of new cases in Canada. The disease was obviously being spread by people who showed no signs of Covid and therefore weren't being tested. The only way to control the spread was to test everyone. Without universal testing the continued—in fact, exponential—transmission of the disease was impossible to prevent.

The role that asymptomatic and presymptomatic people played in keeping the pandemic going wasn't understood until early 2021, when worldwide testing showed that up to 40 percent of people testing positive for Covid-19 exhibited no symptoms of the disease. Many of those had Covid antibodies, which meant they had had Covid-19 and recovered from it without even knowing they'd had it. Virologists recommended social distancing measures to control the spread, but in many countries, politicians worried about the economy (and their popularity) avoided mandating safety measures, keeping retail outlets and restaurants open or reopening them before the spread was under control.

For example, in mid-May 2020, Dr. David Williams, then Ontario's chief medical officer of health, reported that the daily number of new cases from community transmission in Ontario remained stuck in the 200 range, which he considered high, and said he would not recommend an easing of restrictions on store openings until community spread numbers were "well below" 200 new cases daily. On May 17, however, when 341 new cases were reported in the province, Premier Doug Ford relaxed restrictions anyway. In mid-January 2021—when the second wave was in full stride, Ontario had had more than 250,000 confirmed Covid cases, and that number was increasing by more than 2,000 a day—Ford reluctantly mandated a return to restrictions. By then, community spread was up to 84 percent of new cases.

In India, according to the *Hindustan Times*, within a week of the discovery of the Omicron variant, up to 70 percent of new cases were in patients who were asymptomatic, and Delhi's health minister told the newspaper that 46 percent of cases sampled had no history of travel. This indicated community spread.

Realizing that a contagion has become "uncontrollable" is indeed a turning point, not just for epidemiologists but also for the public at large. For health authorities, it means the strategies they've been applying haven't worked and they're back to square one. But worse than that (because square one wasn't that far back), it erodes public confidence in the ability of health authorities to detect Covid in people who don't show symptoms. This in turn leads to a reluctance on the part of the public to follow epidemiologists' next recommendations, and it gives politicians more confidence in ignoring the advice of their own health authorities.

In the November 2020 issue of *The Atlantic*, Dr. Thomas R. Frieden, the director of the CDC during Barack Obama's administration, stated outright that "the coronavirus is growing out of control" and that the incoming Biden government could bring it in line only by implementing "a one-two punch" that would stop the disease from proliferating beyond the reach of medical science. As the first punch, Frieden advocated shutting down parts of society—but strategically, rather than everywhere and all at the same time. Imposing lockdowns on areas that were not highly infected, he said, meant that when the virus eventually did reach that part of the country, people would be fed up with lockdowns and more likely to resist mandated restrictions. The second punch, he said, was universal testing and isolation. Community spread was driven by asymptomatic carriers, and the only way to trace that spread was to test everyone. The goal, he wrote, was to "rebuild social cohesion and trust in one another, and in our government." The title of his article, however, was less optimistic: "We Know How to Beat Covid-19. We Just Don't Do It."

Reproduction Number / (R_o, pronounced "R naught"). *A calculation borrowed from demographics that indicates how contagious a disease is by determining the average number of people, in an uninfected population, who will contract the disease from one person who has it.*

A reproduction number is loosely calculated from a variety of disparate factors, including scientific experimentation, forensic investigations, complex mathematical modeling, and, in many cases, educated guessing. But it does provide a useful measure of comparison among infectious diseases. The R_o of the 1918 influenza virus, for example, was around 1.8, which means that ten people with the flu infected eighteen others, who then infected thirty-two others, and so on exponentially until, in nine generations of the virus (about four or five weeks) those ten cases had become a thousand. If Covid-19 were left on its own, its R_o would be between 2.0 and 3.0. But in tightly confined places, such as school dormitories, high-density apartment complexes, and cruise ships, the R_0 could be much higher. A week after the Covid outbreak on the *Diamond Princess*, the coronavirus's R_0 was 5.7.

A high R_0 does not necessarily mean that the virus is more dangerous. The R_0 of measles is 12, and that of chicken pox is between 10 and 12, whereas the R_0 of smallpox, a much more serious disease than either measles or chicken pox, is between 3.5 and 6. The R_0 of Ebola is only 1.5. The R_0 of common influenza is 0.9 to 2.1, that of SARS is 2.2 to 3.6, and that of MERS is less than 1.

The reproduction number for any disease is an average. On February 13, 2020, researchers in China reported that although in some areas the R_0 for Covid-19 was as high as 6.7, the average for the country was around 2.5, which was bad enough: 1,000 cases became 150,000 cases in about sixteen days. That April, in the United States, Covid-19's R_0 was also 2.5, and that month the WHO declared that 2.5 was the world average. Basically, that meant that the contagion was spreading very rapidly in more places than it was not.

When the R_0 drops to 1, the number of new cases remains steady—one infected person infects one other person. By June 8, 2020, in Ontario, when the first wave was in retreat, the virus's R_0 dropped to 0.8, which meant that ten infected persons infected only eight others. In February 2021, during the second wave, the R_0 rose to 2.2, more or less the same as for SARS. By July, after the third wave, the R_0 had again dropped to 0.84. Only in Alberta, British Columbia, and New Brunswick was it higher than 1 (1.1, 1.1, and 1.3, respectively).

The Delta variant ramped up the coronavirus's R_0 again. By the fall of 2021, Delta's R_0 was between 5 and 6. In November 2021, when Omicron effectively replaced Delta as the dominant variant, studies in both South Africa (where Omicron originated) and Denmark found that the transmission rate for Omicron was more than four times that of Delta's. Omicron and its subvariants BA.1 and BA.2 seemed to be here to stay.

Asymptomatic / *Having Covid-19 but showing no symptoms associated with it.*

On average, a person infected with the ancestral strain of SARS-CoV-2 does not show symptoms for 4.2 days (for subsequent variants, the incubation time can be up to a week) during which time they are termed "presymptomatic"; if, after that, they still show no symptoms, they are asymptomatic. Both conditions pose serious dangers for community spread, as the infected person may not know they are infectious, and their paths through the population are impossible to trace. Early in the pandemic, it was assumed that asymptomatic and presymptomatic persons could not spread the virus, since that had been the case with SARS-CoV-1. As a result, testing for Covid-19 was carried out only on people displaying symptoms.

But as Jonathan Flint writes in the *London Review of Books* on May 6, 2021, "there was published evidence of transmission occurring between people with no apparent symptoms as early as the end of January [2020]." Flint had been part of a group of physicians, geneticists, and computational biologists gathered at UCLA to address the question of asymptomatic transmission. At the time, the state of California hadn't carried out a single virus test, and in the entire country only sixteen people were being tested a day—all of them people who showed signs of having Covid.

"The need to increase the rate of testing," writes Flint, "became urgent when we realized that the virus was spreading between asymptomatic people." Virus tracking had shown that more and more new outbreaks had resulted from community spread, leading researchers to conclude that the disease could only have been transmitted by asymptomatic and presymptomatic persons. Later, the WHO estimated that in some places as many as 80 percent of new cases could be asymptomatic, although in most locales the figure was between 10 and 30 percent.

SARS-CoV-2 is a clever virus. People with Covid-19 who show no symptoms or only mild symptoms benefit the virus because they remain in the general population, providing the virus with maximum covert opportunities for transmission. There is some evidence that virus evolution selects for this form of dissemination: Elisa Gabbert, in *The Unreality of Memory*, writes that a study conducted in 2010 "found that people became more sociable in the forty-eight hours after they were exposed to the flu virus, the period when they are contagious but not symptomatic." Before they started showing symptoms, influenza patients went out more and felt more in need of close contact with others. That may explain why during the pandemic some people so strongly resisted stay-at-home advisories and lockdowns: the virus was urging them to go out and infect more hosts.

In February 2020, when Covid-19's reproduction number was around 4, the number of people infected should have doubled every six days. In fact, cases doubled every three days, meaning the disease was being passed on not only by people who could be identified and tracked, but also by people who would not have seen the need to stay home from work or avoid bars and crowded restaurants.

When the second wave hit in September 2020, universal testing was finally recognized as the best way to manage the pandemic. In Canada, by June 2020, only 47,487 people per million population had been tested; by the end of February 2021, that figure had risen to 696,895 per million, or nearly 70 percent of the total population. Even though the country was in the midst of a second wave, only 3.7 percent of those tested had been positive.

The importance of universal testing became even clearer when, in January 2021, a worldwide study conducted by Scripps Research and published in *Annals of Internal Medicine* found that fully one-third of all those infected with Covid-19 were asymptomatic. A second, more detailed study, published in the *Journal of the American Medical Association* in December 2021, gathered data from ninety-five studies conducted in Asia, Europe, North and South America, and Africa between January 2020 and February 2021. This study found that 60 percent of Covid cases in people under twenty years old were asymptomatic; 50 percent of those between twenty and twenty-nine were asymptomatic; 32 percent between forty and fifty-nine were asymptomatic; and 23 percent of those over sixty were asymptomatic.

The virus revealed many things that were wrong with our society and its infrastructures, chief among them how little we know about genomes, which are the very basis of biology. But we did learn fairly quickly that until vaccines became universally available, the only effective way to control the spread of Covid-19 was to separate people who were infected, symptomatic or not, from the general population, and the best way to do that was to keep everyone home and lock everything down.

That, of course, is exactly what we didn't (and probably couldn't) do.

Covid Toe / *An inflammation of the toes or fingers, similar to chilblain, thought by dermatologists to be a symptom of coronavirus in young patients who are otherwise asymptomatic. Thus a possible diagnostic tool for Covid.*

In March 2020, the husband of New York journalist Jessica Lustig tested positive for Covid-19. Early in his illness, Lustig's teenaged son, CK, who had shown no symptoms of Covid, developed red lesions on his toes. "One day," Lustig reports in the *New York Times* (April 16, 2021), "I said, 'Oh, your shoes are too tight. They must be rubbing you because you have a blister on each toe.' But it turned out to be Covid toes, which is a common symptom among young people. CK still has them."

The inflammation had been reported just that month in Spain by a group of dermatologists who had formed an association called Teledermasolidaria to consult with patients by telephone who were unable to travel to clinics because of Covid restrictions. The doctors had noticed that they received more complaints about chilblain in toes and fingers than usual. Whereas they might have seen ten cases a year before the pandemic, suddenly they were seeing dozens each week.

Chilblain is an inflammation of the blood vessels in reaction to cold and is normally seen in temperate climates during the winter. These symptoms were showing up in warm weather, in Spain, and persisting longer than normal chilblain.

"Over recent days," Nerea Landa, of Teledermaso-lidaria, reported in the *International Journal of Dermatology*, "a series of cases in Spain have begun to emerge" that they believed could be considered a valid reason to administer further tests for Covid-19. Red or purple blisters appeared on patients' toes, heels, or ankles and continued to darken until the lesions formed blisters, the blisters broke, and the condition eventually disappeared "without requiring any treatment." Most patients fell into two groups, with a median age of either thirteen or thirty-one.

After eight months of debate among virologists, however, no direct link between Covid and Covid toe was detected. In January 2021, the *International Journal of Infectious Diseases* reported that although "positive anti-SARS-COV/SARS-COV-2 immunostaining on skin biopsy of chilblains seem to confirm the presence of the virus in the lesions," those same patients continued to test negatively for Covid. A link between Covid and the chilblains, authors Marie Baeck and Anne Herman concluded, was "impossible to confirm."

It may be that Covid toe is just another in the suite of puzzling manifestations of coronavirus infection, along with "brain fog" and loss of smell. The presence of viral particles in the lesions of Covid toe suggests that the condition emerges in the later stages of the infection. But most patients with Covid toe are young and have not had other symptoms, leading some dermatologists to think that the condition is an antiviral immune response, which is how young immune systems respond to a thickening of the capillary walls.

At any rate, Covid toe is not contagious or painful and usually disappears within ten to fourteen days. As Baeck and Herman concluded, more testing is needed.

Polymerase Chain Reaction (PCR) Test / *The standard test used to determine whether a person has Covid-19.*

To administer a PCR test, a health-care worker pokes a long swab up the testee's nose, inserting it into the nasopharyngeal area, the sensitive part of the throat that opens up behind the nostrils. The eerily unpleasant sensation (in Australia, PCR tests are called "brain ticklers") tells us that nothing is supposed to be up there; it's a weak spot in our body's defense against insects. As a result, we have to check ourselves from sneezing. But the ordeal is brief. The swab absorbs mucus, which is then inserted into a reagent that extracts genetic material from the sample. That material is then placed in a tube to react with other reagents that multiply, or "amplify," the sample by making millions of copies of any viral DNA or RNA contained in it. Thus, even a small amount of viral genetic material in the sample will, when amplified, be easily detectable.

PCR tests differ from serology tests; in the latter, a person's blood is tested for the presence of antibodies that the body has produced to defend against an earlier viral infection. Serology tests are less reliable than PCR tests because antibodies may take days or even weeks to develop after an infection. They do, however, show whether a person has been infected with Covid-19 in the past. PCR tests tell whether a person has Covid-19 at the time of testing. PCR tests also differ from rapid antigen tests (or RATs), which test for a particular protein found in coronaviruses. RATs can be purchased in drugstores or online (some governments provide them free) and give positive or negative results in fifteen to twenty minutes.

Mass testing for Covid was slow to get under way for a number of reasons. One was that health authorities thought at first that only people exhibiting symptoms needed to be tested. But a second reason was simple unpreparedness: there weren't enough test kits available. In April 2020, the US was testing 150,000 people a day—a small number considering that Germany, with a tenth the population, was conducting almost the same number. Of those tested in the US, about 20 percent were positive. According to the WHO, that percentage needed to be below 12 before restrictions should be lifted. Dr. Ashish Jha, faculty director at the Harvard Global Health Institute, calculated that to get positive cases down to acceptable numbers, the US would have to test 500,000 people a day every day for a month. Donald Trump assured everyone that was possible, but state governors across the country disagreed, saying they couldn't increase the test rate because they didn't have the materials they needed.

Why was the US so unprepared for a pandemic that had been predicted for more than a decade? The answer is that the predictions came from scientists (and some novelists), and Donald Trump never listened to scientists (or novelists).

Barack Obama renewed the President's Council of Advisors on Science and Technology (PCAST) in April 2010. The council had been formed in 1957, when it was called the President's Science Advisory Committee, by Dwight Eisenhower after the Soviet Union launched Sputnik. Obama asked the council to produce a report on what needed to be done to prepare for a pandemic. On August 19, 2010, PCAST gave him a document called the "Report to the President on Reengineering the Influenza Vaccine Production Enterprise to Meet the Challenges of Pandemic Influenza." In a press release, Harold Varmus, who as a PCAST cochair oversaw the report, stated that "delays involving traditional methods for making influenza vaccines slowed production of a protective vaccine during the 2009–2010 H1N1 influenza pandemic." In what seems now to have been a prophetic statement, Varmus said that "in a serious pandemic, cutting even a few weeks off the vaccine production schedule can translate into saving thousands of lives."

By way of contrast, on January 22, 2017, the morning after his inauguration, Trump dismantled PCAST, had its website removed from the internet, and, to be on the safe side, deleted the council's thirty-nine research papers from public access; he erased PCAST from history. The advisory body remained vacant until October 2019, when Trump began appointing new members to it. The new members, however, were not scientists; they were from industry, and their mandate was to advise the president on how the US could compete with China and Russia for industrial supremacy in the future.

In April 2020, when the pandemic arrived in the US, Trump denied the existence of the pandemic playbook and claimed that the Obama administration had left him with an empty national stockpile. "The cupboard was bare," he said. "You've heard the expression, 'the cupboard was bare.' So we took over a stockpile where the cupboard was bare."

In fact, the stockpile was full. The only items in short supply were N95 face masks, which had been depleted in 2009 during the swine flu outbreak. In 2018, the *Washington Post* reported that the cupboard contained $8 billion worth of medical supplies. If all the supplies in the stockpile had been laid out, they would have covered more than thirty-one football fields. Nevertheless, the masks used during the swine flu epidemic had not been replaced. In 2011, Obama had requested $655 million to replenish the stockpile, but the Republican-led Congress reduced that to $534 million, which meant a decision had to be made between replacing face masks or buying medicine, and medicine won.

Trump's dismantling of PCAST was more than just a dismissal of the role of scientific evidence in political decision making. As Jeffrey Shaman, an epidemiologist at Columbia University, told *Nature* on October 5, 2020, "This is not just ineptitude, it's sabotage." Trump's reactionary views were part of a groundswell of anti-science, anti-intellectual, anti-elite sentiment in the US that has surfaced periodically, arguably since the days of Andrew Jackson, the wealthy, slave-owning president who campaigned as the champion of the common man. The gap has been widening since the days following the Kennedy administration. Being "anti-science" became respectable under "misunderestimated" George W. Bush, who famously announced that "the jury is still out on evolution," and blossomed under Donald Trump, who refused to allow the Environmental Protection Agency to use science-based evidence when calculating its budget.

Like anti-vaccination, anti-science was connected to the religious right, which saw science as an attempt to either improve on the work of God or disprove the existence of God altogether. In Canada, former prime minister Stephen Harper, an evangelical Christian, eliminated the position of national science adviser in 2008, and, as Marci McDonald writes in *The Walrus* in 2006, installed "a point man for the religious right, among other groups, in his government, under the title 'director of stakeholder relations.'" For Harper, science undermined his faith-based policies against abortion and same-sex marriage. For Bush, and later for Trump, science was always pointing out the lunacy of their public pronouncements. Trump's war on science wasn't ideological; it was based on his need to remain in power. Jeff Tollefson, in *Nature*, on October 5, 2020, writes that according to former White House coronavirus task force member Olivia Troye, Trump "repeatedly derailed efforts to contain the virus and save lives, focusing instead on his own political campaign."

Being anti-elite doesn't necessarily mean celebrating stupidity. And yet it so often does. In June 2020, when Covid cases in the US were surging, Trump hastened to assure the public that the apparent increase was not real; it was only the result of an increase in testing. In other words, too much science. "Testing," he tweeted on June 15, "makes us look bad." At a rally in Tulsa, Oklahoma, he told admirers that he had asked his people "to slow the testing down." And at a press conference later that month, he said, "When you test, you create cases."

On September 22, 2021, President Biden announced the appointment of thirty "distinguished leaders in science and technology" to a resuscitated PCAST. Most of the appointees were scientists, and for the first time half of them were women, and a third were immigrants and people of color. Of the three cochairs, two were women: Dr. Frances Arnold, a biochemical engineer and former Nobel laureate; and Dr. Maria Zuber, a geophysicist and planetary scientist who headed nearly a dozen NASA missions.

Biden has been criticized for failing to fulfill his campaign promise to "follow the science" on issues such as mandating vaccinations and making booster shots available to US citizens (he has since made booster shots available to all adults), but as Anthony Fauci, the president's chief medical adviser (who, as director of the National Institute of Allergy and Infectious Diseases, was the scientist most often ridiculed by Trump), told the medical website STAT in September 2021, Biden "made it clear that he wants everyone in this administration, including the medical team, to make sure that science drives the guidelines. That science drives the decisions."

In January 2022, in response to the Omicron surge, the Biden administration announced that every American household would be sent four rapid antigen tests. Similarly, the Australian government promised to distribute 60 million RATs through local pharmacies. RATs are about 85 percent accurate in detecting Covid—less than PCR tests—but they can be given at home and show results in fifteen minutes, as opposed to twenty-four to forty-eight hours. And a study at Johns Hopkins Medicine suggests that RATs and PCRs are equally accurate for children.

Lockdown / *A term originally referring to extreme measures taken to prevent prison inmates (and more importantly, information) from leaving or entering areas where a riot or other disturbance had occurred. During the pandemic, the term was applied to enforced stay-at-home mandates and closures of retail stores, schools, restaurants, offices, and theaters—wherever people might gather in close contact and spread the disease.*

In a somewhat delayed response to an outbreak of what was then called pneumonia, on January 23, 2020, the Chinese government imposed "the Wuhan lockdown" on the city in Hubei province in which Covid was first detected. The WHO called the lockdown "unprecedented in public health history." By January 24, the lockdown—and the disease—had spread to the entire province of Hubei. All public transport was halted, and no one was allowed to leave the city—although advance notice of the lockdown allowed 300,000 people to flee Wuhan before the 10 AM deadline. After that, only one person in each household was allowed to leave the house every two days. The restrictions remained in place until April 8. By then, 3.9 billion people worldwide—half the population of the Earth—were living under some form of lockdown.

Even before the pandemic, the term "lockdown" had expanded beyond its militaristic context. But it was usually associated with violence and crime. For example, US airspace was placed on "lockdown" after 9/11, and the city of Boston was locked down after the Boston Marathon bombing in 2013. So it may be that when Covid hit, the word "lockdown" already had a negative, restrictive connotation in the public imagination, which might partly explain why there was so much resistance to it.

Susan Sontag, in *Illness as Metaphor*, her book about how the meaning of "cancer" has metastasized beyond the field of medicine, traces the use of military terminology to describe medical phenomena to the 1880s, a few decades after Louis Pasteur developed the germ theory of disease: a germ was an enemy that could be fought and subdued. The late nineteenth century was a particularly bellicose period in European history, and its metaphors tended to be militaristic. With the discovery of microbes, medicine became a war between diseases on one side and patients on the other. "Bacteria were said to 'invade' or 'infiltrate,'" Sontag writes, like an invading foreign army.

In this century, applying military terminology to any sort of endeavor, strenuous or not—we've had the War on Poverty, the War on Drugs, the War on Terror—is common and somewhat disheartening, because none of those wars appear to be winnable. The terms persist because they give the appearance of determination and organization: dealing with terrorism as an ongoing campaign does not require us to look into the social and political causes of terrorism, just as treating disease as an enemy does not require us to examine the social and political causes of disease. Military or criminal terms are regularly applied to Covid-19: we have an "invasion" met with "frontline workers" who are "heroes," and a mounting "body count." Vaccines have been developed that "target Covid-19."

Early in the pandemic, Trump declared that "we want to finish this war," adding that "this is an all-out military operation that we've waged." In April 2020, US surgeon general Jerome Adams said, "This is going to be our Pearl Harbor moment, our 9/11 moment." It might have been more accurate to say it was America's Vietnam moment, or its Desert Storm moment: an all-out offensive against a largely unseen and poorly understood enemy that constantly eluded detection.

In *The Plague*, published in 1947, Albert Camus reversed the military metaphor by using a medical term to stand for a military situation. In the novel, the plague that rapidly contaminates Europe is a metaphor for the spread of Nazism. In a copy of the novel Camus gave to his friend Jacqueline Bernard, he wrote, "To J., survivor of the plague." "This was a reference," writes Bernard, "to my recent return from a German concentration camp." Camus referred to restrictions made necessary by the disease as "a kind of imprisonment," a sentiment readily shared by many who endured stay-at-home orders during the Covid pandemic.

When we talk about a disease as if it were a tangible enemy that can be defeated by waging war against it, we open the door to measures put in place to suspend civil liberties and human rights, and give governments extraordinary powers. As the *Washington Post* observed, "the specter of 'war'... has prompted unhelpful forms of panic, cleaning out store shelves and—in the United States—leading to a troubling rush for guns." In 2020, gun shops in the US reported a 65 percent increase in sales over 2019, and that rush to arms continued in 2021. "Sales usually spike around elections," the *New York Times* noted on May 29, 2021—which is in itself alarming—but never by so much. "Americans have been on an unusual, prolonged buying spree fueled by the coronavirus pandemic, the protests last summer, and the fears they both stoked." American gun shops sold more than a million guns per week, one-fifth of them to first-time owners. As Los Angeles city councillor Marqueece Harris-Dawson told the *Times*, "Americans are in an arms race with themselves." The proliferation of gun sales alone should have encouraged more people to observe the lockdowns.

In Canada, Prime Minister Justin Trudeau told Parliament in April 2020 that the pandemic is not a war. "There is no front line marked with barbed wire, no soldiers to be destroyed across the ocean, no enemy combatants to defeat." What we had was a medical emergency; the disease needed to be treated, the afflicted comforted. As the Spanish ambassador to the US, Santiago Cabanas, told the *Washington Post* in March 2020, "there is a temptation to use war terms.

We don't need weapons, we don't need bombs. We need solidarity and compassion."

Apart from places like China, Australia, and Argentina—citizens of Buenos Aires were kept in continuous lockdown for more than two hundred days—most countries imposed closures and stay-at-home measures sporadically and for short periods: two weeks here, a month there. The idea was to curtail the spread of Covid-19 until the number of new cases appeared to be lessening and then to open up businesses before the economy tanked. As a result, both a nation's health and its economy suffered in alternating fits and starts.

In Margaret Atwood's post-apocalyptic novel *The Heart Goes Last*, when the American economy collapses in "a big financial-crash business-wrecking meltdown," Stan and Charmaine volunteer to participate in a social experiment in which they live relatively normal, productive lives in a controlled community called Consilience for one month. They are then transported into total lockdown in a prison called Positron for a month and then go back to Consilience, and so on, presumably forever. Part of the agreement is that, as in *The Handmaid's Tale*, the couple can't back out and can have no contact with the outside world.

As the novel's title suggests, the experiment doesn't end well. Prisoners almost always find ways to circumvent a lockdown.

Self-Isolation /

"Impossible, I realize, to enter another's solitude."
PAUL AUSTER, *The Invention of Solitude*

Self-isolation is the act of secluding oneself from all contact with others to lower the risk of spreading or catching a disease. Originally a reference to a country's foreign policy—as in, "China's self-isolation policy during the Qing dynasty led to economic stagnation"—the phrase is now commonly used in popular psychology. Pam Garcy, the author of The Power of Inner Guidance, *notes that "people with depression are notorious for self-isolation."*

During the pandemic, people have been encouraged, and sometimes ordered, to self-isolate. Ottawa Public Health refers to self-isolation as "when you are sick with symptoms of Covid-19 and you have been told by a health care provider or Public Health to separate yourself from others." However, even people without symptoms of Covid-19 self-isolate voluntarily, reducing their contact with others, especially strangers, to avoid being infected with coronavirus.

Psychological treatises from the Before Times indicate that self-isolation is not always a good thing. A 2017 study conducted at Brigham Young University by psychologist Julianne Holt-Lunstad found that social isolation can produce negative health effects equivalent to smoking fifteen cigarettes a day or having a serious drinking problem. "Being connected to others socially is widely considered a fundamental human need," says Holt-Lunstad. "There is robust evidence that social isolation and loneliness significantly increase risk for premature mortality." In the midst of a pandemic, too much contact with others can kill you, but so can too much isolation.

Holt-Lunstad's study and others like it examined the effects of long-term self-isolation among vulnerable populations over years, but the European Public Health Alliance warns that there are also risks associated with shorter periods of social isolation, as occasioned by Covid, and policy makers should consider these risks when issuing stay-at-home orders. "The impact of isolation and loneliness should not be under-estimated or fall to the bottom of politicians' lists of priorities," cautioned the Alliance, "as inaction now will lead to high human and financial costs later on." After spending time in isolation, some people never want to come out of it.

Isolation has profoundly negative effects on brain function, both psychological and physiological. Catherine Offord, writing in *The Scientist* (July 13, 2020), cites studies showing that prolonged terms of isolation and loneliness are linked with cognitive decline, dementia, increased memory loss, and premature mortality. She notes that in 2018, when the nine-person crew of the Antarctic research station Neumayer III returned from a fourteen-month stay at the South Pole, MRIS performed before and after the stay "showed anatomical changes to the dentate gyrus, a region of the brain that feeds information into the hippocampus and is associated with learning and memory." The crew members' dentate gyruses had shrunk by nearly 7 percent. Their blood also had lowered levels of brain-derived neurotrophic factor, a protein that helps to regulate stress and memory. "And they performed worse on tests of spatial awareness and attention."

At the time, the tests were designed to assess the possible effects of long-term space travel; since the pandemic, however, psychologists are looking at these and similar tests to determine how we as individuals and as a society may be affected by periods of long-term self-isolation due to Covid.

For those whose separation from the outside world is both prolonged and unrelieved—who may feel like prisoners in an isolation cell—the long-term effects may be profound. Instead of depression causing a sense of self-isolation, self-isolation can produce depression and anxiety. A neighborhood newspaper in the city where I live ran a story recently about a local artist who had moved to the city to take a job at Queen's University. "Then the pandemic hit, and everything changed." When restrictions "put a halt to everything," the artist found herself working from home, "feeling isolated and struggling with her mental health." As she told the paper, "I felt a little shorted." She was, however, able to turn to art to relieve her feelings of depression and anxiety.

Others may not have that outlet. Conspiracy theorists to whom I have spoken, some of whom genuinely believe that the pandemic is a government plot and that vaccines contain microchips that will make us all more controllable, are generally single, spend a lot of time on the internet, and live much more secluded lives than most of us. Their self-isolation, partly enforced, partly circumstantial, may make them more susceptible to superstition and paranoia. An article in *Scientific American* published in May 2017, titled "Conspiracy Theorists May Really Just Be Lonely," reported on an experiment conducted by Princeton psychologist Alin Coman, in which subjects were asked to write about an unpleasant social interaction they'd had with friends and then to rate their belief in two conspiracies (one, that the government uses subliminal messages to control behavior, and two, that pharmaceutical companies withhold cures so that people will continue to spend money on treatments). "The more excluded people felt," writes Matthew Hutson, the article's author, "the greater their desire for meaning and the more likely they were to harbor suspicions."

The current pandemic has made a lot of people feel lonely.

In a review of two novels about women who habitually isolate themselves—Rachel Cusk's *Second Place* and Jhumpa Lahiri's *Whereabouts*—Claire Dederer writes that both novels' narrators "seem to have freed themselves of the familiar forms of wanting."

Perhaps, in our separate fastnesses, some of us have learned not only to want different things, but also to want things differently.

Social Bubble / *A small group of family members and/ or close friends permitted to associate without masking or social distancing during periods of lockdown.*

In a piece published on April 28, 2020, Canada's *National Post* observed that "Canadians have been living in bubbles," adding that the word "bubble" "sounds non-scientific, vaguely frivolous... and a bit silly," but "is actually a powerful tool of pandemic response enforcement."

"Bubble" was first applied to the pandemic in New Zealand, one of the earliest countries to restrict social movement, when Prime Minister Jacinda Ardern told families who were chafing at being cooped up in their houses that they could "slightly extend [their] household bubble, but keep it local, small and exclusive." She meant that one household could bubble with one other household. The idea was to allow people some relief from lockdown, but not enough to cause another wave of Covid.

In April 2020, New Brunswick permitted "two-household bubbles," or "double bubbles," similar to those in New Zealand. Newfoundland followed suit in May. According to New Brunswick's guidance document, double bubbling "would allow you to visit, have a meal and enjoy the company of another household bubble. You must not have close contact with anyone else. You cannot join up with more than one household or bubble." Soon, bubbling became common across Canada and the US and in many European countries. In July 2020, when the UK eased lockdown restrictions, the government allowed healthy travelers to holiday in sunny locations like Spain without having to undergo quarantine or isolation on their return; these trips were termed "travel bubbles," a comforting notion, perhaps, but actually the opposite of bubbling with one other household.

Forming a social bubble with another person or group was called a powerful tool of pandemic response because it allowed people to live in relative safety without suffering overmuch from isolation. Writing in *The Atlantic* (May 28, 2020), epidemiologist Julia Marcus notes that the government of the Netherlands encouraged people who were in quarantine to find themselves a *seksbuddy*—a designated sexual partner—to prevent them from spreading the coronavirus by seeking multiple partners. The US government, she says, remained silent on ways that Americans could stay mentally and physically healthy during lockdowns, leaving people with no options other than life as usual or total self-withdrawal.

Policies in the Netherlands and Canada, says Marcus, focused on "harm reduction" rather than "abstinence only." The harm-reduction model is better because "people will take risks" (remember Nick Paumgarten's "we are nothing if not weak") and without guidelines for resolving the many practical dilemmas involved with isolation, they'll take unnecessary and possibly dangerous risks, such as gathering in large groups in parks and on beaches. "The oft-cited concern," she writes, "is that offering people strategies to reduce the harms of risky behavior will end up *promoting* that risky behavior." For example, offering drug users clean needles and safe injection sites was thought to encourage more people to use drugs. Even though studies clearly show that it doesn't, assumptions linger.

Choosing bubble mates within a family caused friction in times that were already tense. Parents with more than one adult child had to decide which one they were going to stay close to and which they would go without seeing for the unforeseeable future. The media called it a kind of Sophie's choice, a reference to William Styron's novel of that name in which a mother has to choose whether to rescue her son or her daughter from a Nazi concentration camp. Grandparents had to choose not only between their children but also among their children's children. Such choices led to resentment, but more often to heartache and guilt.

But social bubbles also carry risks. Much of the discussion around choosing who to bubble with sounded a lot like selecting a spouse. "Negotiating to become part of someone else's intimate circle in the midst of a pandemic," warns Gideon Lichfield in the *MIT Technology Review* (May 9, 2020), "is fraught with dangers both medical... and social." Lichfield emphasized the importance of choosing one's "quaranteam" carefully: all members must be exclusive, must comply with mandated restrictions, and should probably not work as frontline health professionals. "What you're going into," he writes, "isn't a friendship, but a partnership."

In the United States, when people were allowed to form social bubbles, or "pods," they were also warned that bubbling could be dangerous if it wasn't strictly controlled. In November 2020, Rachel Gutman pointed out in *The Atlantic* that "the answers to some basic questions—how many people should be in a bubble? what's okay for the members of a pod to do together?—are still unclear." Gutman found that the definition of "bubble" was often loose and leaks were not uncommon. Bubblers she spoke to said their bubbles ranged in size from three to thirty-five members and in some cases extended into the hundreds because of leakages. "As soon as you sort of break your bubble," warned Beth McGraw, of Penn State's Center for Infectious Disease Dynamics, "the connections can be infinite. And this is how [the virus] spreads."

In May 2020, Germany allowed two households to visit one another's homes, and Belgium specified that a household of four could invite four other people to make a "corona bubble." Epidemiologists believed that contact tracing of four guests would be possible. France, Austria, and Denmark allowed social gatherings of up to ten people, which was getting away from the notion of small, containable social bubbles.

Some feared that social bubbling could produce a "filter bubble," a term coined in 2010 to describe the state of intellectual isolation resulting from website algorithms that show users only those sites the algorithm thinks they want to see, based on information gleaned from their previous internet history. People relying on the internet for their information about the real world—as was increasingly the case during pandemic lockdowns—become isolated from sources with different viewpoints, and so their biases are rarely challenged.

This is similar to the "echo chamber" effect, in which beliefs are amplified or reinforced by communication and repetition inside a closed system—for example, the military—creating a "confirmation bias." The filter bubble phenomenon has been linked to Trump's success in the 2016 presidential campaign, during which Russian hackers are believed to have flooded US voters with pro-Trump propaganda. In Barack Obama's farewell speech, he warned that "a retreat into our own bubbles" could pose "a threat to democracy."

Rebecca Solnit maintains that the alt-right in the US is living in a political bubble. In her essay "Whose Story Is This?" she recounts that in March 2018, "*PBS*

NewsHour featured a quiz by Charles Murray... that asked 'Do You Live in a Bubble?'" The quiz posed such questions as "Have you ever walked on a factory floor?" and "Have you ever had a close friend who was an evangelical Christian?" PBS failed to mention, Solnit writes, that Charles Murray was "widely considered a racist." Murray was the coauthor of the 1994 book *The Bell Curve*, in which he asserted that Black people in the US consistently scored lower than white people on IQ tests (a review in *Scientific American* called the book an "endorsement of prejudice").

The PBS quiz, writes Solnit, "was essentially about whether you were in touch with working-class small-town white Christian America" and implied that if you were not, then you weren't a true American. She writes that "the quiz delivered the message, yet again, that the 80 percent of us who live in urban areas are not America." In other words, about 80 percent of Americans live in an elitist bubble. Solnit turns that around, saying that "the actual problem is that white, Christian, suburban, small-town, and rural America includes too many people who want to live in a bubble and think they're entitled to." That would be about 20 percent of Americans, or 70 million people, roughly the number who voted for Donald Trump.

Transmission Unit / *Any person who may infect another with coronavirus; in other words, anyone.*

"Among the many things that Covid-19 has upended," writes storyteller and social activist Annie Tan in a blog post in April 2020, "it has changed the way we express and experience love. When each person and family becomes a possible 'transmission unit,' celebrations, communal rituals and gatherings increasingly seem like a careless way of putting those you love most at risk."

In July 2021, when Ontario's anti-Covid restrictions were gradually being lifted, our son and his family, who live in Toronto, came to visit us. We had seen them only twice in the previous eighteen months, always outside, wearing masks and keeping social distance. This time, with cases in our city down to almost zero and all of us double-vaccinated, we felt we could selectively relax our vigilance and expand our social bubble to include them. But our son kept his face mask on. He was not afraid of contracting Covid from us; he worried that we might contract it from him. We respected his wish to follow the Covid protocols until the pandemic was over, but his actions made us realize how frightened some of us had become at the thought of being transmission units.

In Emily St. John Mandel's post-apocalyptic novel *Station Eleven*, published in 2014, she envisions a world that has been reduced to scattered oases of survivors following a viral pandemic known as the "Georgia

Flu." Like SARS-1, the Georgia Flu killed its victims rapidly—and spread so thoroughly that within a year the world's population had been reduced by more than 90 percent.

Early in the novel, Mandel gives "an incomplete list" of the many things the survivors miss about their lives "before the collapse." Among them: "No more diving into pools of chlorinated water lit green from below. No more ball games played out under floodlights . . . No more certainty of surviving a scratch on one's hand, a cut on a finger while chopping vegetables for dinner, a dog bite. No more flight. No more towns glimpsed from the sky through airplane windows, points of glimmering light; no more looking down from thirty thousand feet and imagining the lives lit up by those lights at that moment . . ."

One of the things she might have added to the list: no more spontaneous, uncomplicated holding of our children or grandchildren in our arms.

Pivoting / *Switching to a business model that will get a company through the pandemic and hopefully lead to longer-term growth and security when the pandemic is over.*

The term "pivot" has been around for a long time. I learned to pivot playing high school basketball—you start running in one direction until blocked by an opponent, then you spin around and take off in a different direction. In business parlance, "pivot" describes what start-ups do when, after starting up, they find that the reality of the marketplace differs from what they had expected and have to quickly switch to an alternate business model. Often, a plan B is already in place as a backup.

With the pandemic, however, even companies that had been operating for years suddenly found themselves having to come up with new strategies in order to avoid bankruptcy, and they often didn't have a plan B on hand. They had to scramble. But scrambling isn't pivoting. In basketball, you pivot to a clearer path toward the basket. In business, a successful pivot extends the company's existing abilities, aligns with the specific conditions created by the pandemic, and introduces new ideas that the company can continue to use when the pandemic is over.

For example, many restaurants that only offered indoor dining before the pandemic set up tables on sidewalk patios. Some also offered curbside pickup, or home delivery, or both. Others opened small boutiques inside their doors, in which they sold precooked frozen food, olive oil, flowers, candles, and other meal-related items. One restaurant in our city changed the designation on its window from "ristorante" to "food and wine shop." If pivoting saw them through the mandated restrictions, some continued to offer these services after health authorities allowed them to reopen. Similarly, local farmers who had previously been delivering their produce to restaurants began delivering directly to customers' homes, and advertising their services—such as weekly preorders and menus—on online platforms such as Shopify.

In "How Businesses Have Successfully Pivoted During the Pandemic," the *Harvard Business Review* gives examples of several large companies that underwent "a thorough transformation" during the shutdowns, not only to deal with the crisis but also to prepare for eventual recovery. Before the pandemic, Spotify made music available to many users for free and disproportionately relied on advertising for income. During the pandemic, when advertisers either disappeared or else cut back on their ad budgets, Spotify began to offer original content in the form of podcasts produced in collaboration with artists. Users responded by uploading 150,000 podcasts in the first month, so Spotify signed exclusive deals with many artists and celebrities, effectively becoming the copyright holders of those podcasts, much as Netflix owns the rights to its in-house television series.

Airbnb is another company that pivoted successfully during the pandemic. Actually, it pivoted before the pandemic, too. It started out in 2007 as a small company in San Francisco that rented air mattresses to visiting business travelers who couldn't find hotel rooms. That quickly led to helping those same conference goers find accommodation in private homes.

Until Covid hit, the company wasn't much more than a website that matched hosts with guests (although its estimated worth was around $38 billion), but when restrictions on travel came into effect, hosts and guests became scarce. In 2020, Airbnb began "Online Experiences," a full-range lifestyle platform that included online cooking classes, virtual bicycle and hiking tours, music and travel features, and other programs to keep travel alive in people's minds during the pandemic and give them new ideas and places to explore once the crisis was over.

In the post-pandemic world, Airbnb executive Catherine Powell told *Fortune* magazine in September 2020, "people are going to need to connect and want that social interaction." Although people will feel "less tethered," she said, Airbnb's pivot showed that "you can actually connect incredibly personally and emotionally" in a virtual setting.

Large hotels, especially those in cities, had a different problem. Most of them made the bulk of their profits from hosting sizable gatherings—weddings, conventions, annual general meetings—and those were precisely the kind of events to which Covid put an end. Accommodations experts estimate that major hotels in India, for example, lost 75 percent of their revenue in 2020. The Indian Hotels Company Limited alone, one of the country's biggest chains, reported a loss of 7.96 billion rupees in 2021. "The Covid conundrum," writes Chumki Bharadwaj in *India Today* on

July 14, 2021, "with its successive waves, has been particularly harsh."

While some hotels, like the Hyatt Mumbai, shut down completely, others pivoted in unique ways. Some hotels owned by the ITC chain partnered with local hospitals to offer quarantine facilities for asymptomatic and mildly symptomatic patients. The LaLiT Mumbai went so far as to offer vacation packages to guests that included a free vaccine—until, that is, the government pointed out that it was illegal to sell vaccine doses. Including vaccines in an all-inclusive package doesn't qualify as a pivot, anyway, because it isn't something that would be continued when the crisis is over.

Flatten the Curve / *Attempt to slow the spread of Covid-19 by mask-wearing, handwashing, and social distancing so that the number of Covid-19 cases requiring hospitalization doesn't overwhelm health-care facilities.*

The phrase first appeared on March 9, 2020, on an illustrated graph designed by microbiologist Siouxsie Wiles and artist Toby Morris for The Spinoff, a New Zealand online publication. The graph, entitled "Flatten the Curve," shows two mound-like curves, one rising and descending steeply and the other rising slowly, peaking at a lower level but lasting longer.

The image part of Morris's graph was based on a previous graphic included in a 2007 CDC publication entitled "Interim Pre-pandemic Planning Guidance: Community Strategy for Pandemic Influenza Mitigation in the United States." The CDC graph showed both curves and noted that social distancing and keeping children home from school would help to prevent cases from surpassing hospital capacities in the event of an eventual pandemic, which it predicted would hit the world within five years. The Spinoff graph resembled the CDC graph, but the addition of the title drove home the difference between the two mounds. In both curves, the same number of people became sick and entered hospitals, but with the flattened curve the impact was spread out over a longer period of time, meaning that there would be no sudden, overwhelming demand on limited facilities and staff—and fewer deaths.

Perhaps because of the easy-to-understand graphics, the phrase was quickly picked up by health authorities urging people to exercise caution. As early as March 15, Dr. Anthony Fauci, the director of the National Institute of Allergy and Infectious Diseases (NIAID), told reporters that "if you look at the curves of outbreaks, they go big peaks, and then come down. What we need to do is flatten that down." To do that, he said, Americans might have to go into a national lockdown.

Harnessing the two phrases—"flattening the curve" and "national lockdown"—got people's attention. Politicians wanting to appear that they knew what they were talking about used the phrase "flattening the curve" to pat themselves on the back. In Ontario, for example, Premier Doug Ford, under pressure after bobbling the ball in the early stages of the pandemic (as almost all right-wing leaders around the world did), assured the public on October 6, 2020—the end of a week that had seen an average of 611 new Covid-19 cases a day, compared with 125 a month earlier—that "we... flattened the curve." By January 2021, one-quarter of all ICU beds in Ontario were occupied by Covid-19 patients, and more than half of the province's ICU units were filled to capacity.

From early in the pandemic, flattening the curve with nonpharmaceutical interventions such as lockdowns, face masks, and social distancing was intended to reduce the number of daily new Covid cases and relieve pressure on overwhelmed ICUs in countries around the world. In January 2021, when vaccines became available, a new goal was added: to flatten the curve by vaccinating as many people as possible. In the US this was important because, as Nicholas Christakis points out in *Apollo's Arrow: The Profound and Enduring Impact of Coronavirus on the Way We Live*, "the United States has fewer hospital beds per capita than other industrialized countries; the US has 2.9 beds per 1,000 people, whereas South Korea has 11.5, Japan has 13.4, Italy has 3.4, Australia has 3.8, and China has 4.2." It didn't take many severe Covid cases to overwhelm the American health-care system;

whereas India ran out of oxygen, the US ran out of beds. Gradually, stepping up vaccination rates relieved the pressure on the health-care system. In August 2021, Johns Hopkins infectious disease expert Amesh Adalja told Vox that in countries where the vaccination rate was 40 percent or higher, "what we've seen is a decoupling of cases and hospitalizations."

And so, the rush to develop vaccines and get them into as many arms as possible, as quickly as possible. In the US, only one-fifth of the hospitals are run by the government; the rest are either privately owned not-for-profits (58.4 percent)—which rely on fees for service, insurance coverage, and donations—or frankly for-profit establishments (21.3 percent) which are given tax breaks for offering a certain amount of charity work for their communities (such as walk-in vaccination clinics), which costs them a lot less than paying taxes would. These are the establishments that, when Covid struck, quickly ran out of face masks, gowns, ventilators, and beds. The first goal of flattening the curve, of course, was to save lives—but how good would it be if US hospitals could save lives and save money, too?

Herd Immunity / *The hoped-for state in which a population is immune to an infectious disease.*

On September 15, 2020, when the US had mourned more than 200,000 deaths from Covid-19, Donald

Trump maintained that the pandemic would end on its own, without science and with no mandated interventions by federal and state governments. During an ABC News town hall, Trump told host George Stephanopoulos that Covid-19 would eventually just "disappear."

G.S. Without the vaccine?

D.T. Sure, over a period of time. Sure, with time it goes away—

G.S. And many deaths.

D.T. And you'll develop—you'll develop herd—like a herd mentality. It's going to be—it's going to be herd-developed, and that's going to happen.

The gaffe highlighted Trump's tenuous grasp on the reality of the pandemic. "Before you start wearing what everyone else is wearing just to make the virus disappear," wrote Bruce Y. Lee in *Forbes* the next day, "keep in mind that Trump most likely meant 'herd immunity.'" I'm not sure Lee was right. It's possible that Trump really did think that a herd mentality might save his presidency, that if people just shut up and did what he said, the pandemic would simply go away. He certainly seemed to have believed that later, after the 2020 presidential election.

Herd immunity is the utopia of pandemic philosophies. How attractive the concept that if we simply do nothing, the disease will eventually go away. The belief is based on the assumption that a person who recovers from a contagious disease will have developed a natural immunity to that disease, by virtue of the antibodies produced by the immune system. Early in this pandemic, the attraction of herd immunity was based on the assumption that Covid-19 behaved like other viral infections. Smallpox, for example: a person who survives smallpox will in all likelihood not contract it again.

But even if that were true for Covid-19, it's hard to fathom how anyone could advocate allowing a highly contagious respiratory disease to run unchecked through a population in the hopes that the survivors would be immune. In any case, it isn't true for Covid: getting it once does not mean you won't get it again.

Attempts to reach a state of herd immunity with Covid have taken two opposite, though not mutually exclusive, routes. By route A, which mandates the complete lockdown of bars, restaurants, retail outlets, schools, and international borders and issues stay-at-home orders to everyone, we allow the disease to run its course through the population until everyone who is going to get it has gotten it and either recovered or died. Route B is the complete absence of any restrictions whatsoever, combined with eventual universal vaccination, until the great majority of the population is either naturally or artificially immune. Authorities differ as to how great that majority needs to be, but 70 to 80 percent is the usual figure.

Neither approach worked. Route A, which was tried in China, Hong Kong, New Zealand, and Australia, for example, kept the number of new cases down and bought time for the development of vaccines but risked the ire of the population and the collapse of the economy. Route B allowed the economy to stagger on, but risked high numbers of infections and deaths. Medical professionals almost universally advised route A; politicians generally took route B. Some governments— Canada, the US, and most of Europe—experimented with a seesaw route between A and B, which ensured that neither was traveled long enough for the results to be conclusive.

In late 2020, advocates of the no-restrictions-just-let-us-party-on school received unexpected support from the American Institute for Economic Research, a libertarian think tank located in Great Barrington, Massachusetts, that claims to be nonpartisan but publishes treatises with titles such as "Biden's Tax Plan Is a Middle-Class Death Tax Dressed as a Capital Gains Tax on the Rich" and "What Greta Thunberg Forgets About Climate Change" and posts ads on social media denouncing the use of face masks and social distancing. In October 2020, the institute issued its "Great Barrington Declaration," which declared that herd immunity is the only way to beat Covid-19 and that governments should stop mandating restrictions and just let the pandemic run its course. "We know that all populations will eventually reach herd immunity," it read, without saying how they knew that. "The most compassionate approach that balances the risks and benefits of reaching herd immunity, is to allow those who are at minimal risk of death to live their lives normally to build up immunity to the virus through natural infection, while better protecting those who are at highest risk. We call this Focused Protection."

Twelve thousand people signed the Declaration. At least as many called it ill-informed and dangerous. Stephen Archer, head of the Queen's University Department of Medicine, called it a "cognogen," an infectious, bad idea. In a rebuttal published in The Conversation in November, Archer listed a number of reasons why the Declaration should be ignored. For one thing, by denouncing mandated restrictions and advocating unlimited personal freedom, the Declaration placed personal freedom above the public good. For another, it didn't specify how it would "better protect" vulnerable populations. Most damning of all, the Declaration "misunderstands herd immunity." In the US, there had been 9 million cases of Covid, and fewer than 10 percent of Americans had antibodies in their systems. Saying that people who had had the disease should be allowed to mingle freely with those who hadn't, he said, "amounts to a global chicken pox party." The Declaration did little other than provide fodder to "the 19 percent of North Americans who don't trust public health officials," and to the 40 percent of eighteen- to twenty-four-year-old Americans who, as of December 2021, still weren't vaccinated.

The point at which a high enough percentage of the population has been vaccinated against an infectious disease—or developed enough immunity through infection—that the disease goes into retreat is called the "herd immunity threshold." With highly infectious diseases—measles, for example—the threshold is reached when 80 to 90 percent of the population is immune. At that point, the likelihood that an infected person will come into contact with someone who is still susceptible to the disease is low enough that the disease does not spread. For Covid-19, the threshold is between 70 and 80 percent. Without widespread vaccination, reaching that threshold takes time—possibly centuries—and so waiting for herd immunity is not an ideal strategy for eliminating a rapidly mutating viral infection such as Covid-19.

Although vaccines against Covid-19 were developed in record time, a significant percentage of the population in developed countries still refuse to get them, and as of January 2022, most developing countries were unable to procure enough doses to vaccinate even 5 percent of their citizens. In many of those countries, vaccine hesitancy has been a mitigating factor. And recent studies show that recovering from Covid-19 does not confer lasting immunity; some suggest that the antibodies produced by the body's immune system remain in effect for only a few months, after which a person is once again susceptible to the disease, which has been the thinking behind recommendations for multiple doses, or boosters.

Early in the pandemic, Swedish health authorities urged social distancing and the wearing of face masks but allowed businesses and restaurants to remain open to keep the economy flowing. No one used the term "herd immunity," but that was the strategy they were using. They gambled that 80 percent of the population would contract Covid-19 and develop antibodies faster than pharmaceutical companies would develop, test, and release vaccines. By the end of April 2020, 7.3 percent of Stockholm citizens tested for Covid-19 were positive, a figure not significantly higher than that of other countries that had gone into early lockdown. By June, however, Sweden had 37,000 confirmed cases, more than all the other Nordic countries combined, and more deaths per capita (5.29 per million per day) than any other country in Europe.

By February 2021, Sweden's Covid death rate was still higher than that of any other Nordic country. Denmark, Norway, and Finland, with a total population of 16.75 million, had recorded 3,763 deaths; Sweden, with a population of 10.3 million, had had 12,826 deaths. The figures prompted some observers to say that Sweden's herd immunity policy had been a bad plan. However, more than half of Sweden's deaths were patients in long-term care facilities, and a further 25 percent were over seventy years of age and being cared for at home. A lockdown of the entire population probably would not have lowered the death rate among that elderly vulnerable population. This was felt to be encouraging evidence that herd immunity hadn't been such a disaster after all.

But it had been. In March 2021, in a letter to the editor of the *New England Journal of Medicine*, Yoshiyasu Takefuji of Keio University, Japan, compares Sweden's Covid record with that of Taiwan. Herd immunity did not come out looking good. "Taiwan," writes Takefuji, "implemented a robust 'digital fence,' using mandatory coronavirus apps to isolate asymptomatic and presymptomatic carriers of [Covid-19] and to prevent contact with uninfected persons." Sweden, with its population of 10.3 million, had had 10,185 deaths by January 14, 2021; Taiwan, with a total population of 23.8 million, had had only seven deaths.

In China, it appeared for a while that border closings, complete lockdowns, and mass vaccination might lead to herd immunity. In March 2021, China was administering about 5 million vaccinations a day; this increased to nearly 20 million doses a day, and by early June more than 600 million Chinese citizens had been vaccinated. "Some Chinese experts now say," writes Vincent Ni in *The Guardian* , "that the country is on its path to achieving 'herd immunity.' " But 600 million in a country of 1.4 billion is still below the herd immunity threshold for Covid, and those 600 million people had been given a Chinese vaccine that had a low effectiveness rate. "The virus won't go away," stated public health expert Yanzhong Huang, "and perhaps it's time to update our thinking on the so-called 'herd immunity'... Ultimately, we need to live with the virus."

In the UK, the debate about herd immunity versus lockdown was not so much a debate as a policy swap. As James Butler writes in the *London Review of Books* (April 16, 2020), herd immunity (through widespread infection as opposed to eventual vaccination) was part of the British government's model, devised in 2011, for dealing with a possible influenza outbreak—and was simply hauled out and dusted off when the coronavirus showed up. On March 1, Patrick Vallance, the UK's chief scientific adviser, told Radio 4 that one of the "key things we need to do [is] build up some kind of herd immunity." The government delayed switching to lockdown for twelve days, until computer modeling showed that a herd immunity approach could result in as many as 250,000 deaths. Meanwhile, the delay had allowed the virus to spread extensively: Paul Garner, an infectious diseases professor who became sick during those twelve days, refers to himself as a member of "the Boris Johnson herd immunity group."

Is there a herd immunity threshold for Covid? On October 19, 2021, the UK registered 44,000 new cases, the highest number of new cases in one day since January, even though 80 percent of its population was fully vaccinated.

The big problem with herd immunity, apart from the fact that it doesn't work for Covid-19, is a moral one. Allowing the disease to spread unchecked, or only partially checked, virtually condemns a large and identifiable portion of the population to death. In October 2021, the *New York Times* reported that the Brazilian senate tried to have President Jair Bolsonaro charged with "crimes against humanity" for allowing Covid-19 to spread along the Amazon among people opposed to increased logging, "in a failed bid to achieve herd immunity and revive Latin America's largest economy." In Canada, people with compromised immune systems and those over the age of seventy accounted for more than 80 percent of Covid deaths. Isolating vulnerable people (in long-term care facilities, for example) in the hope of achieving herd immunity in the rest of the population is not immunizing the herd; it's culling it.

3

Vaccines and Miraculous Cures

"The question is not how to get cured,
but how to live." JOSEPH CONRAD

Hydroxychloroquine / *A drug used to treat patients with rheumatoid arthritis or lupus; championed by Donald Trump and others as an effective treatment for Covid-19.*

"And the hydroxychloroquine is a—I hope it's going to be a very important answer," said Donald Trump on April 4, 2020. "We're having some very good things happening with it, and we're going to be distributing it through the Strategic National Stockpile. It's going into the Strategic National Stockpile to treat certain patients. And we have millions and millions of doses of it; 29 million to be exact."

Such high hopes for hydroxychloroquine were based on an isolated experiment conducted at a university in France in which in vitro injection of the drug into a coronavirus appeared to prevent the viral particles from replicating. White House enthusiasm for the treatment waned, however, when six patients in clinical trials in Brazil died, indicating that hydroxychloroquine was dangerous to anyone with a heart condition. The French trials could not be replicated in other labs and were deemed "meaningless" by medical professionals. In late May, France prohibited doctors from prescribing it. Despite these results, under pressure from the White House, the Food and Drug Administration gave hydroxychloroquine Emergency Use Authorization, and in Brazil, hydroxychloroquine and chloroquine—an antiviral drug sold for cleaning fish tanks—were subsequently approved to treat coronavirus patients in hospitals.

The same month, Donald Trump admitted he had been taking "the hydroxy" for a week and a half. Met with criticism from health professionals, he replied, "All I can tell you is so far, I seem to be okay." Which prompted comedian Jimmy Kimmel to observe, "Our president is a hydroxymoron."

In June, the FDA revoked its Emergency Use Authorization for both hydroxychloroquine and chloroquine, "based on recent results from a large, randomized clinical trial in hospitalized patients that found these medicines showed no benefit for decreasing the likelihood of death or speeding recovery." A month later, however, a new study, conducted by the Detroit-based Henry Ford Health System, suggested that hydroxychloroquine was an effective treatment for coronavirus after all, and the White House (and therefore Fox News) put renewed pressure on the FDA to reinstate the drug's Emergency Use Authorization.

Dozens of studies showed that hydroxychloroquine conferred no protection whatsoever against Covid-19, and even Trump backed off from promoting it. When Trump contracted Covid-19 in October 2020, he was given a wide variety of treatments, including monoclonal antibody injections, zinc, melatonin (to regulate his sleep patterns), famotidine (for heartburn), remdesivir, and vitamin C—but, perhaps significantly, no hydroxychloroquine. Even Fox News stopped talking up the drug.

In November, *The Lancet* published the results of a huge trial conducted by Christopher Rentsch, an epidemiologist at the London School of Hygiene & Tropical Medicine who specializes in "creating real-world evidence for the safety and effectiveness of medications." Since hydroxychloroquine was commonly prescribed to patients with systemic lupus erythematosus and rheumatoid arthritis, Rentsch wondered if patients who had been receiving hydroxychloroquine since before the pandemic were less susceptible to Covid-19 than people who had not. He examined the records of 30,569 rheumatoid arthritis and lupus patients who started taking hydroxychloroquine six months before the pandemic and compared them with 164,068 patients with the same conditions who had not been treated with hydroxychloroquine. "Taken together," he wrote, "our findings do not provide any strong support for a major protective effect from ongoing routine hydroxychloroquine use."

Even so, health professionals in the US called for more tests, noting that the drug had been used for various conditions since the 1960s and was safe. Finally, in February 2021, virologist Bhagteshwar Singh and four colleagues reviewed fourteen studies that investigated the effectiveness of hydroxychloroquine either as a preventative or as a treatment for Covid-19, and Singh reported to Cochrane, a UK-based international health research network, that "hydroxychloroquine is not beneficial for patients with Covid-19 who require care in hospital. The evidence is less clear for prevention of Covid-19 and for people being treated as outpatients. However, with no benefit when used for treatment of severe Covid-19, a benefit in these situations is unlikely."

To this, one coauthor added, "This review certainly should put a line under using this drug to treat Covid-19, but some countries and health providers are still caught up in the earlier hype and prescribing the drug. We hope this review will help these practices end soon."

It did.

Monoclonal Antibodies / *Antibodies made by cloning white blood cells in a lab. The cloned blood cells produce antibodies that are then injected into a patient to fight off the infection.*

The monoclonal antibody injections given to Donald Trump when he had Covid-19 in October 2020 were developed by the biotech company Regeneron. Trump called the treatment a "cure" and promised the experimental drug to anyone who needed it, free of charge. Regeneron, however, had only 50,000 doses and said it would be able to produce only a few million more, raising the uncomfortable question of who would be chosen to receive Trump's miracle cure.

Eli Lilly and Regeneron each produced two antibody therapies that were very effective in combination but not alone. In February 2021, the FDA approved the use of Eli Lilly's combination of bamlanivimab and etesevimab for patients who were in the early stages of infection and who were not on oxygen or ventilators. In March, however, the company halted distribution of bamlanivimab because new coronavirus variants proved to be unaffected by it.

Meanwhile, other pharmaceutical companies were producing their own monoclonal antibodies. A Russian biotech company, BIOCAD, developed a treatment it claimed prevented the excessive production of inflammatory proteins (cytokines) that were the cause of the "cytokine storms" that overwhelmed patients' immune systems. Although approved in Russia, no other country accepted the treatment because BIOCAD would not publish its test data.

An Indian company, Biocon, developed a treatment that also worked against cytokine storms by targeting specific molecules on the cell surface that regulate the immune system. The therapy was approved in India, but not elsewhere, because its clinical trial had included only thirty patients.

Interest in monoclonal antibody therapies declined when vaccines became available, but revived in July 2021, when the Delta variant spread across the US and cases again began spiking. States with large numbers of vaccine-hesitant people, like Texas, Tennessee, and Florida, opened monoclonal antibody treatment centers as alternatives to vaccination centers, and Florida governor Ron DeSantis called the therapy "the best thing we can do to reduce the number of people that require hospitalization." In Tennessee, Fox News reported that monoclonal antibody infusion therapy was "continuing to see success." The article quotes Dr. Lisa Piercey, Tennessee's department of health commissioner, saying that the treatment "very likely could prevent hospitalization or even death."

Immunologists remained skeptical of such claims. There was a strong scientific backlash in October 2021, for example, when Regeneron's cofounder and chief scientific officer, George Yancopoulos, told an audience in Boston that an infusion of monoclonal antibodies might have saved the life of Colin Powell, the former secretary of state, who had died of complications from Covid earlier that week at the age of eighty-four. Yancopoulos claimed that his company's treatment could have saved not only Powell, but up to 80 percent of the

Americans who had died of Covid. Epidemiologists agreed that monoclonal antibodies provided some relief from symptoms in people who already had Covid, especially in those who were immunocompromised and could not produce antibodies of their own, but the FDA has not approved the treatment for general use.

There are those with weakened immune systems or comorbidities for whom vaccinations are either not an option or not sufficient protection against the coronavirus. For such patients, AstraZeneca produces a monoclonal antibody treatment called Evusheld, designed specifically for immunodeficient patients, to be administered before exposure to Covid. Tests showed that Evusheld reduces the risk of Covid by 80 percent and that the treatment remains effective for up to six months. The US and Canadian governments both gave the treatment authorization for emergency use in January 2022. Depending on how "immunocompromised" is defined, between 3 and 14 percent of North Americans have compromised immune systems.

Carvativir / *Another supposed miracle drug, this one hailed by Venezuelan president Nicolás Maduro as both a preventative and a treatment for Covid-19.*

In a Facebook video posted by Maduro (and subsequently taken down by Facebook), the Venezuelan president promoted Carvativir as the *gotas milagrosas*—miracle drops—that were an alternative to vaccines to prevent infection by coronavirus. "Ten drops under the tongue every four hours," he said, "and the miracle is done." Developed by "a brilliant Venezuelan mind," Carvativir would both prevent and cure Covid-19. When Facebook froze Maduro's page, following WHO guidelines against misinformation about the pandemic, Maduro continued to promote the product on other social media accounts and called Facebook's action "digital totalitarianism."

Maduro did not name the brilliant mind who had developed Carvativir, but the *Washington Post* identified him as Raúl Ojeda, a medical researcher working for Labfarven, the Pharmacological Laboratory of Venezuela.

In Mexico, my wife and I put a drop or two of oil of oregano under our tongues when we feel a cold or the flu coming on. It tastes awful but seems to work at least as well as any over-the-counter cold remedy—and is one herbal solution that shows some experimental efficacy. We buy it from a shop in San Miguel de Allende. The shop is lined with dark wooden shelves full of ceramic pots with signs and symbols on them that make us feel we are buying an ancient folk remedy—which we are. The main compound of oil of oregano is carvacrol, a compound also found in large quantities in marjoram, Mexican oregano (*Lippia graveolens*), and dittany of Crete (*Origanum dictamnus*), which has been used as an herbal remedy since at least the time of Homer.

The similarity between the names Carvativir and carvacrol suggests a possible basis for Maduro's claim. Carvacrol, also known as isothymol, is a compound found in traditional remedies that treat respiratory ailments and gastral disorders. In Virgil's *Aeneid*, Venus treats Aeneas's wounds with dittany, an herb "not unknown... to wild goats, when winged arrows have lodged in their flank." A study published in May 2020 in LitCovid—a curated literature hub for scientific information about Covid-19 published by the US National Library of Medicine—found that isothymol derived from *Ammoides verticillata*, a member of the family that includes carrots and parsnips, acts as an inhibitor to angiotensin-converting enzyme 2 (ACE2), which is the receptor through which the coronavirus enters host cells.

Although it's possible that Carvativir, whatever it is, is effective in warding off viruses, promoting it as an alternative to vaccines is the kind of political obfuscation in which Trump engaged when he pimped for hydroxychloroquine. The truth is that the United States imposed economic sanctions on Maduro's socialist government, and although food and medicines were exempt from those sanctions, Jorge Arreaza, Maduro's foreign minister, told the *Washington Post* that businesses and banks were reluctant to help Venezuela buy vaccines in case they drew the ire of the US president. "No bank will receive Venezuelan money," said Arreaza, "for fear of sanctions." Maduro had to come up with a homegrown treatment for Covid, and Carvativir was at hand.

Ivermectin / *A drug designed to treat parasites in animals and river blindness and elephantiasis in sub-Saharan Africa, but widely promoted as a treatment for Covid-19.*

The codiscoverers of avermectin, the parent drug of ivermectin—William Campbell and Satoshi Ōmura—were awarded the Nobel Prize in Physiology or Medicine in 2015 for their work on the treatment of parasitic diseases. Although ivermectin was sold by Merck (where William Campbell was employed) to treat heartworm in livestock, in 1987 the company began distributing it at no cost for the treatment of river blindness. In subsequent studies, it turned out that in very high doses it is also an effective antiviral agent against RNA viruses such as SARS-CoV-2. But the doses required to treat coronaviruses are too high to be safely ingested by humans.

In May 2020, before vaccines were available, ivermectin was promoted by Brazilian president Jair Bolsonaro as a cure for Covid-19. That April, a paper had been published by the preprint server Research Square claiming that a study conducted in Egypt showed that the drug reduced Covid-19 death rates by more than 90 percent. That paper was retracted when a graduate student at the University of London read it and realized he had read some of it before, in other papers. Further investigation turned up dozens of patient records that appeared to be duplicates of each other, records of people who had died before the study began, and numbers that looked a little too convenient.

However, "before its withdrawal," notes Sara Reardon in *Nature* in August 2021, "the paper was viewed more than 150,000 times, cited more than 30 times and included in a number of meta-analyses that collect trial findings into a single, statistically weighted result." It was like the MMR vaccine to autism connection a decade earlier. By the time the paper was discredited, ivermectin had been seized on by conspiracy theorists on social media as a weapon against Covid that the powers that be were keeping to themselves.

In the US, the FDA posted a warning with the unambiguous title, "Why You Should Not Use Ivermectin to Treat or Prevent Covid-19." The FDA specified that "certain animal formulations of ivermectin such as pour-on, injectable, paste, and 'drench,' are approved in the US to treat or prevent parasites in animals." The drug is sold in farm supply stores to treat diseases in horses caused by worms. "For humans," the FDA said, "ivermectin tablets are approved at very specific doses to treat some parasitic worms, and there are topical (on the skin) formulations for head lice and skin conditions like rosacea." The FDA, however, "has not authorized or approved ivermectin for the treatment or prevention of Covid-19 in humans or animals."

This disclaimer, of course, was taken by conspiracy theorists as proof that ivermectin was a miracle cure. As someone posted on the Facebook group Ivermectin vs. Covid, "Ivermectin is clearly the answer to solve covid and the world is waking up to this truth." According to the *New York Times*, the watchdog group Media Matters for America found sixty public and private Facebook groups dedicated to sharing information about ivermectin. Facebook closed down twenty-five of them, but the remaining thirty-five had a total of nearly 70,000 members.

In South Africa, where the drug is banned for human use, an anti-vax group called South Africa Has a Right to Ivermectin (SAHARI), which also has 70,000 members, has demanded that the drug be prescribed for Covid. Ivermectin, claims SAHARI, is a "medication that has proven to have a positive effect on Covid-19 and other illnesses, such as the Zika virus." In the US, hospitalizations from ivermectin poisoning tripled in 2021 over 2020: 1,440 cases were treated in the first eight months of the year. In New Mexico, two people died after taking ivermectin. In Pennsylvania in February 2022, a doctor was fired from a hospital run by the Tower Health Medical Group for prescribing ivermectin.

"It's hard to understand why people would turn down an FDA-approved Covid preventative in favor of a treatment that's not only unapproved but has a large body of evidence showing it doesn't work," pediatrician Nathan Boonstra told NBC News in August 2021. "But anti-vax groups will eat up any opportunity to make it seem like a vaccine isn't needed."

NBC also reported on advice posted by a Reddit user, warning that "even if you can get an Rx for IVM, the pharmacy may not fill it for 1–3 days claiming they don't have it in stock, which is pure bulls——." And which is why, advised the user, you should always "HAVE SOME HORSE PASTE ON HAND."

Remdesivir / *A broad-spectrum antiviral drug, developed by Gilead Sciences to treat hepatitis C and Ebola. Also known as Veklury.*

Remdesivir failed when tested against Ebola in 2014, but later showed promise in preventing the MERS coronavirus from replicating. Early in the pandemic it was tested in Wuhan as a treatment for Covid, with inconclusive results: about the same number of people died after taking remdesivir as died in the placebo group.

A second trial, conducted by the National Institute of Allergy and Infectious Diseases (NIAID) in the US, was three-quarters through when patients who had been given remdesivir showed an improved mortality rate—8 percent died, compared with 11.6 percent in the placebo group. NIAID immediately directed researchers to stop the trial and start giving remdesivir to all patients, saying it was unethical to withhold the drug from those in the placebo group. The FDA awarded the drug Emergency Use Authorization, which meant it could be used in hospitals and clinical trials but could not be prescribed to the general public.

Remdesivir received approval in the US on October 8, 2020—the first treatment for Covid to receive FDA approval—for patients over twelve years of age who had Covid and required hospitalization. Soon, more than half the Covid patients in the US were being treated with the drug. A study published in the *New England Journal of Medicine* on November 5, 2020, found that remdesivir did seem to have some benefits: hospitalized patients with Covid receiving the drug showed shorter recovery time (ten days from admittance, as opposed to fifteen days in a placebo group), lower mortality (6.7 percent compared to 11.9 percent after fifteen days), and fewer side effects. Nonetheless, on November 20, the WHO "recommended against" its use, stating there was "no evidence that remdesivir improves survival and other outcomes." On July 15, 2021, a study reported on the medical news site Medscape found no Covid survival benefits related to remdesivir. Gilead disputed the study's findings but eventually canceled remdesivir's clinical trials when vaccines became available.

In May 2022, *The Lancet* published the findings of a trial conducted from March 22, 2020, to January 29, 2021, by the WHO Solidarity Trial Consortium. For the study, 8,275 patients, who were selected from sixty-five countries in all six WHO regions and who were already hospitalized with Covid-19, were randomly given either doses of remdesivir or no drug at all. At the end of the trial, it was found that 19.6 percent of those who had been given remdesivir died, and slightly more— 22.5 percent—of the control group had died. The study authors concluded that remdesivir "has no significant effect on patients with COVID-19 who are already being ventilated. Among other hospitalised patients, it has a small effect against death or progression to ventilation (or both)."

In countries where vaccine doses are in short supply and Covid cases are piling up, treating patients with remdesivir offers them a slightly better chance of recovery. And, as Nicholas Christakis notes in *Apollo's Arrow*, shortening the length of hospital stays, even by a day or two, relieves pressure on overburdened healthcare systems. When new Covid cases surge, as they do with each new variant, "freeing up ICU capacity is a crucial objective."

Molnupiravir / *An oral antiviral drug developed in pill form as a treatment for Covid-19.*

Merck, partnered with Ridgeback Biotherapeutics, began human trials with molnupiravir in October 2020 and applied to the FDA for approval a year later.

The trials seemed to go well, and in June 2021, the US government placed an advance order for 1.7 million courses of the treatment, on condition that the drug received Emergency Use Authorization from the FDA, which it received in December. It has also been approved in the UK. It has not been approved in Europe. Although Canada has bought half a million courses, saying it will buy a further half million if Health Canada approves the treatment, by mid-June 2022 approval for the drug had not been forthcoming.

Four capsules are taken twice a day for five days, meaning a single course of treatment requires forty capsules. As of October 2021, a single course cost seven hundred dollars, although Merck said it planned to implement a sliding price scale so poorer countries could afford to finance their health responses to the pandemic.

Molnupiravir works by introducing errors into the coronavirus's genetic code that cause the virus to mutate so much, it can't replicate. In a press release, Merck claims that the drug reduces hospitalizations by 30 percent and lowers the number of deaths in patients who already have Covid. The idea is that a drug like molnupiravir would be highly beneficial in a country where vaccines are unavailable and treatment by monoclonal antibodies, which requires injection, is impractical.

Merck warns that molnupiravir is toxic to human fetuses, making it dangerous for women who don't know they're pregnant. Pfizer also advises pregnant women not to take Paxlovid without consulting their doctors.

Paxlovid / *An oral antiviral therapy for Covid-19 consisting of two drugs: nirmatrelvir and ritonavir, administered within five days of a patient testing positive for Covid.*

The *New York Times* reported in November 2021 that Pfizer expected to come out with an oral Covid treatment called Paxlovid by the end of the year. The treatment consists of thirty pills taken over five days, and treatment must be commenced within five days of developing symptoms. Pfizer claimed that in clinical trials, Paxlovid reduced hospitalizations and death by 89 percent, and the US government promptly ordered 10 million courses of treatment (thirty pills per course). In January 2022, they committed to buying another 10 million courses, for free distribution to US patients twelve years and older at high risk of being hospitalized with Covid. Pfizer committed to providing the first 10 million courses by the end of June 2022, and the second 10 million by the end of September. On January 17, 2022, Canada approved Paxlovid for immunocompromised patients eighteen years and older.

The three pills taken twice daily are two of nirmatrelvir and one of ritonavir. Nirmatrelvir inhibits the enzyme that the Covid virus needs to make more copies of itself within human cells, thereby essentially ending the infection. Ritonavir, a drug originally used to treat AIDS, is a booster for the nirmatrelvir. It also shuts down the metabolism of nirmatrelvir in the liver, so that the drug remains in the body longer and continues to inhibit the virus's spread.

In May 2022, a phenomenon called "Paxlovid rebound" was reported in the medical journals. The claim was that four to five days after the course of treatment with Paxlovid, symptoms of Covid-19 began to reappear in some patients. Pfizer replied that in its clinical trials, rebound was experienced in 5.6 percent of takers, compared to 0.3 percent among those who were given a placebo.

Rachel Gutman, writing in *The Atlantic* on May 26, 2022, points out that the clinical trials carried out by Pfizer were of unvaccinated persons at high risk of contracting Covid, and the drug was tested only against the Delta variant. Gutman writes that doctors she spoke to said that with Omicron, they were seeing Paxlovid rebound in many more than 5.6 percent of their patients. Paul Sax, of Brigham and Women's Hospital, told her that in his view, the number of patients experiencing rebound was "way more than half."

Convalescent Plasma / *Blood taken from a recovered coronavirus patient, reduced to a serum containing a high concentration (or high titer) solution of antibodies, and injected into a patient with early symptoms of Covid-19 to help reduce the risk of further infection.*

In the February 27, 2020, edition of the *Wall Street Journal*, Arturo Casadevall, of the Johns Hopkins School of Medicine, wrote an op-ed piece describing how during a measles outbreak in 1934, a physician extracted blood from a boy who had recovered from measles, and injected it into thirty-four of the boy's classmates. None of them got measles. Casadevall suggested that the same concept could be used for SARS-COV-2.

When Michael J. Joyner, a professor of anesthesiology at the Mayo Clinic in Rochester, Minnesota, read the piece, he contacted Casadevall and proposed they conduct a joint experiment at the Mayo Clinic. Within months, they had tested the technique on 70,000 Covid patients across the US and found that, when the plasma was given within three days of diagnosis to patients under the age of eighty who were not on ventilators, the death rate was 22 percent. In patients four days and longer from diagnosis, the death rate was 27 percent. Although that may seem a small difference, with 70,000 patients, it meant 3,500 fewer deaths.

The study had been designed to test the safety of the procedure, not its efficacy as a treatment for Covid. But

Donald Trump, desperate for good news about Covid before the 2020 federal election in November, hailed convalescent plasma at a press conference in August as a miracle cure, saying it was "proven to reduce mortality by 35 percent." No one knew where he got that figure. Nonetheless, on August 23, Trump demanded that the National Institutes of Health (NIH) approve the treatment for emergency use, which the NIH had already refused to do. Trump then publicly announced that the Food and Drug Administration (FDA) had granted an Emergency Use Authorization for the treatment. As Arthur Caplan observed the next day on the medical website STAT, "the fact that [the announcement] came a day before the start of the Republican National Convention tells a story all by itself."

When confirming the approval at a press conference, FDA commissioner Stephen M. Hahn claimed that if convalescent plasma had been used earlier, 35 percent of those who had died would have recovered—an outrageous, unsupported, and dangerous claim, according to the scientific community, since no clinical trials of the procedure had been carried out. Health officials worried that the approval of convalescent plasma might actually increase the danger of coronavirus by making clinical trials more difficult. As had happened with remdesivir, not giving a drug that appears to be working to a placebo group raises ethical questions.

Early studies of the effectiveness of convalescent plasma on Covid patients in India, conducted in

September 2020, found little or no benefit in the treatment. In the trials, reported in the *British Medical Journal (BMJ)* on October 22, 19 percent of patients who received the plasma treatment "clinically deteriorated or died" within twenty-eight days, whereas 18 percent of patients who received usual care without plasma grew worse or died.

Further studies, however, reinstated convalescent plasma as an effective technique. A paper published in *The Lancet* on March 23, 2021, found that although the treatment was not particularly effective for patients with late-stage Covid-19, it did benefit those in the early stages of the disease. The optimum treatment, the study found, occurred when the plasma was taken from a recovered Covid-19 patient between one and three months of the disappearance of symptoms, when the patient's antibody production was at its peak. Benefits were even greater when the recovered patient had also received the Pfizer-BioNTech vaccine. The authors recommended that the plasma be harvested on the day the patients returned to the clinic for their second Pfizer shot.

The development of successful vaccines siphoned much of the urgency from convalescent plasma research, but the treatment is still recommended for patients in the early stages of Covid-19 who are likely to develop more severe symptoms later. A paper published in the *New England Journal of Medicine* in February 2021 concluded that "early administration of high-titer convalescent plasma against SARS-CoV-2 to mildly ill infected older adults reduced the progression of Covid-19."

Vaccines / *From the Latin* vacca, *meaning "cow," whence* vaccinia, *cowpox, which in nineteenth-century England was also called "the vaccine disease." To "vaccinate" originally meant to inoculate a person with cowpox to prevent that person from contracting smallpox.*

Militaristic metaphors notwithstanding, a vaccine doesn't directly attack a virus. A vaccine tricks the body's immune system into attacking an imaginary virus so that when the real virus comes along, the body is ready for it. It's not unlike the US military sending train-and-equip forces into Afghanistan to prepare Afghan troops to fight the Taliban—except that in the case of vaccines, the strategy works. A vaccine "trains" the human immune system to produce antibodies that will attack the virus. Some of them even teach human cells not to reproduce copies of the invading virus.

A vaccination against Covid-19, then, does not give a person a mild dose of Covid-19. Infecting a person with a small amount of a disease to prevent a more serious case of that same disease is not vaccination; it's "variolation." To vaccinate means to give a person a case of a related but milder disease so that the person's immune system produces antibodies that are effective against the more serious disease.

For centuries, variolation was commonly practiced in Asia and Africa, where parents would give their children a dose of smallpox (by inserting a smear of exudate from another patient's smallpox pustule under the child's skin) so that their bodies would resist the disease later on. The Boston minister Cotton Mather, in a letter published in the *Philosophical Transactions of the Royal Society* in 1714, reported that he heard of the practice from his African servant, Onesimus (a biblical name meaning "useful"), who said that "he had undergone an operation, which had given him something of the smallpox and would forever preserve him from it, adding that it was often used among the Guaramantese [probably Ghanaians] and whoever had the courage to use it was forever free of the fear of contagion."

Variolation was introduced in England in 1721 by Lady Mary Wortley Montagu, who had witnessed the treatment while residing in Turkey. At the time, one of every twelve deaths in England was caused by smallpox. Although variolation worked, it was scary; the medical establishment didn't know how it worked and mistrusted anything coming from a non-European culture, and so it banned the practice. We can imagine the conversation:

"You want to prevent this person from getting smallpox?"

"Yes."

"How do you intend to do that?"

"By giving him smallpox."

Variolation continued to be practiced in the UK, but not by doctors. It remained a kind of folk remedy for the rest of the eighteenth century.

It didn't get less scary after that. In 1796, Dr. Edward Jenner experimented with cowpox, a viral disease similar to smallpox. He took pus from a pustule on the hand of Sarah Nelmes, a dairymaid who had cowpox, and injected it under the skin of an eight-year-old boy, James Phipps, the son of Jenner's gardener. Six weeks later, Jenner injected Phipps with smallpox, and the boy did not develop the disease. Jenner infected Phipps with smallpox twenty more times, with the same result, and Phipps lived to the age of sixty-five. By then, vaccination had been approved as a preventative against smallpox. In 1798, Jenner declared in the *Medical and Physical Journal* that "having suffered the vaccine disease will prove a preservative from the infection of the small-pox." Since then, inoculations against a host of infectious diseases are all referred to as "vaccines."

Covid Vaccines / *The nearly two dozen* SARS-CoV-2–*specific vaccines developed against Covid.*

In developing vaccines against Covid-19, researchers were able to take advantage of work already done on vaccines for SARS and MERS. In fact, it was thanks to those earlier coronavirus outbreaks that many scientists were semi-prepared for the Covid-19 pandemic, if no one else was. Designing a vaccine against an infectious disease usually takes ten to fifteen years. Before Covid, the fastest vaccine development had been for mumps, which took four years; it was five years before a vaccine against Ebola was produced. But since researchers had been working on vaccines against coronavirus infections since the early 2000s, developing a number of highly effective vaccines against the closely related Covid coronavirus took less than a year. As Nicholas Christakis writes in *Apollo's Arrow*, by May 2020, "over one hundred different vaccines of an astonishing variety were already in the works, supported by university laboratories, pharmaceutical companies, and governments around the world. Many of these had entered human trials."

One of those labs was at the National Institute of Allergy and Infectious Diseases (NIAID), located in North Bethesda, Maryland, where Dr. Anthony Fauci presided. One of the NIAID biologists, Barney Graham, had been working on inserting a particular mutation into the protein of a virus so that it would instruct a human cell to produce antibodies. He was originally trying to develop a vaccine against RSV, the virus that causes wheezing pneumonia in children, and when MERS showed up, he realized the technique might also work against coronaviruses. As Lawrence Wright explains in *The Plague Year*, the problem was how to introduce the modified protein to the human immune system. "Graham knew that Moderna, a biotech startup in Cambridge, Massachusetts, had encoded a modified protein on strips of genetic material known as messenger RNA." Within a day of the publication of the SARS-CoV-2 genome sequence on January 11, 2020, Graham and a colleague, Jason McLellan, designed a modified protein that would work for the Covid coronavirus, and on January 13, they handed the modified spike protein over to Moderna. In February, Moderna began advertising for volunteers for clinical trials, and the first human was inoculated with a Moderna mRNA (messenger RNA) vaccine on March 16.

Messenger RNA research has a long and interesting history. Moderna was established in 2010—the name of the company is a mashup of "modified" and "RNA"—to commercialize the research of Harvard biologist Derrick Rossi, who was developing a way to use mRNA as a medical therapy. The company quickly grew after 2013, when it signed a five-year agreement with AstraZeneca to produce an mRNA treatment for cardiovascular diseases. It also researched the application of mRNA delivery platforms for use in vaccines and was in the process of developing two dozen vaccines for clinical trials when Covid appeared on the scene. Before that, the company had had only one drug pass Phase I trials, a treatment for myocardial ischemia, called AZD8601.

In 2017, Moderna began using an mRNA delivery system similar to that developed by the Canadian company Acuitas Therapeutics, started by University of British Columbia biochemist Pieter Cullis, which protected the mRNA in balls of fat to be delivered to the interior of target cells. Acuitas had developed this liposomal or "lipid nanoparticle" (LNP) delivery technology for Alnylam Pharmaceuticals, a Massachusetts-based company that developed a successful treatment for the hereditary disease of transthyretin amyloidosis using small interfering RNA (siRNA) to silence a pathological gene in the liver.

In the meantime, BioNTech, a company started in Germany by two Turkish immigrants to develop mRNA therapies for cancer, had begun working with Pfizer on an LNP mRNA vaccine for influenza using a formulation provided by Acuitas. BioNTech was joined in 2013 by Katalin Karikó, who, while working with Drew Weissman at the University of Pennsylvania, had discovered the secret of preventing the immune system from attacking and destroying mRNA, a discovery that Damian Garde and Jonathan Saltzman, writing in STAT in November 2020, called "the starter pistol for the vaccine sprint to come." In 2020, when the pandemic hit, all efforts were transferred to developing a lipid-wrapped mRNA vaccine for Covid-19.

That year, Moderna's CEO, Stéphane Bancel, promised then-president Trump that Moderna could deliver a Covid vaccine within three months. Trump appointed a Moderna board member, Moncef Slaoui, to be head scientist for Operation Warp Speed, a catch-up initiative set up by Trump to make it look as though he was taking Covid seriously, and Moderna received a $483 million grant to bring its vaccine to market.

In contrast, Albert Bourla, CEO of Pfizer, refused the offer of government money and committed over $1 billion of Pfizer's resources not only to run a large, expedited clinical trial to ascertain the effectiveness of the Pfizer-BioNTech vaccine but also to scale up manufacturing so that millions of doses could be available as soon as the vaccine was approved. This approach was, of course, based on the assumption that the vaccine would be approved; Bourla made a very risky bet on success.

Pfizer's bet paid off when the announcement was made in November 2020 that the Pfizer-BioNTech vaccine was 95 percent effective for preventing Covid, regardless of the age, sex, or ethnic background of the recipient. As a result, on December 11, 2020, the US FDA approved the Pfizer vaccine for emergency use, even though human trials had not begun until May. The Pfizer-BioNTech vaccine was fully approved for use in the UK, the EU, and the US in August 2021. The results obtained for the Moderna vaccine were remarkably similar to Pfizer's and also earned it emergency approval.

It was, however, a different type of vaccine, one produced by AstraZeneca, that was the first to be administered in the UK. Scientists at Oxford University had worked on creating a vaccine against MERS and teamed up with the pharmaceutical company AstraZeneca to produce it. Like Pfizer, AstraZeneca was a seasoned drug manufacturer. Formed in 1999 by the merger of the Swedish pharmaceutical company Astra AB (which produced penicillin and the anesthetic Xylocaine) and the British Zeneca Group (which was known for its cancer-care centers in the US and for the oncological drugs Casodex, Nolvadex, and Zoladex), the merged company was headquartered in London and maintained its research and development and manufacturing facilities in Sweden. Its best-known, and best-selling, product was Crestor, a cholesterol-lowering medication that earned the company $5 billion a year, but for which the patent would expire in July 2021.

The Oxford-AstraZeneca vaccine is viral vector, meaning that it uses a virus that is different from a coronavirus—in this case, it uses the adenovirus that causes the common cold in chimpanzees—to trick the immune system into creating antibodies against coronavirus. AstraZeneca was the first company to publish the results of its Phase III trials and was approved for emergency use in the UK early in December 2020. It didn't get full approval because there was an anomaly in their data; a number of participants in the trial had accidentally been given a half-dose for their first shot instead of a full dose, and for some unknown reason, patients in that group had fared better than those who had received a full dose. Regulators sent back the Oxford-AstraZeneca vaccine for more trials, and the UK approved the Pfizer vaccine.

The Pfizer-BioNTech vaccine (also known as tozinameran, BNT162b2, or by its brand name, Comirnaty) has been approved in eighty-two countries—in some, such as Canada and the US, for vaccinating people as young as six months. It originally required two doses delivered twenty-one days apart and was found in early studies to have an efficacy rate of 95 percent, beginning one week after the second dose. A later study, published in the *New England Journal of Medicine* in September 2021, gave the Pfizer vaccine an efficacy of 89 percent at reducing hospitalizations and death. A UK study also found that Pfizer reduced the probability of contracting Covid-19 in the first place by 80 percent.

The Moderna vaccine (mRNA-1273), approved in forty-six countries—in some, such as Canada and the US, for people six months and older—also requires two doses but was designed to be delivered twenty-eight days apart. It had an efficacy rate of 94.1 percent two weeks after the second dose. The more recent *NEJM* study, published in September 2021, found Moderna's efficacy over a longer period was 96 percent. The main drawback for both the Pfizer and Moderna vaccines was that they had to be stored at –70 degrees Celsius (–94 degrees Fahrenheit), which required refrigeration equipment not available in poorer countries.

Oxford-AstraZeneca, approved for use in ninety-one countries, is given in two doses up to four months apart and is 82 percent effective with a twelve-week interval between doses. In fact, trials suggest that the vaccine is more effective with a longer interval than if the two doses are delivered closer together.

Early in the vaccine rollout, vaccine shortages in some countries forced health authorities to use their entire stock of vaccines to give one dose to as many people as possible. This tended to make the Astra-Zeneca vaccine a better option, since there were no data to say how effective an mRNA vaccine would be beyond their recommended intervals. Research in the UK in January 2021, however, supported a twelve-week interval for AstraZeneca; Oxford University recommended an eight- to twelve-week interval. Twelve weeks gave patients 76 percent protection during the interval, and 84 percent after the second dose. A second study, published in *The Lancet* in February 2021, found that AstraZeneca's effectiveness increased twelve weeks after the first dose, whereas if the second dose was given after six weeks, effectiveness dropped to 55 percent; it was better to wait the full three months between injections.

The US never approved the AstraZeneca vaccine. Canada approved it in February 2021 but advised that the vaccine might not be suitable for people over sixty-five years of age. That advisory was lifted in March. The minimum age for receiving the vaccine was originally fifty-five and has gradually been reduced to eighteen.

The European Commission approved three vaccines—Pfizer, Moderna, and AstraZeneca—although Hungary, along with forty-five other countries, ordered doses of the Russian vaccine Sputnik V. In February 2021, the French National Authority for Health announced that a second dose of any vaccine was not necessary for those who had already had Covid, assuming that people who had recovered from the virus had developed sufficient antibodies on their own and that the first dose was sufficient to provide full coverage against Covid.

Also in February 2021, Janssen Pharmaceuticals, a division of Johnson & Johnson located in Belgium, delivered 80,000 doses of its single-dose vaccine (also known as JNJ-78436735 or Ad26.cov2.S) to South Africa, even though clinical trials had not been completed. The vaccine delivers adenovirus 26 to human cells, provoking the immune system to switch on the cell's alarm bells. The viral vector vaccine was reportedly 66 percent effective in preventing moderate to severe Covid-19 and 57 percent effective against the Beta variant. It has since been approved in forty countries.

In early March 2021, the Johnson & Johnson vaccine was approved for use in the US. Some rural and Black communities rejected it, however, feeling it was less effective than the Pfizer-BioNTech and Moderna mRNA vaccines. As Darrell J. Gaskin, a health policy expert at Johns Hopkins, told the *New York Times*, people felt as though there was "a luxury vaccine and then the non-luxury vaccine." By mid-March, however, the J&J vaccine was considered by many health authorities to be the best choice for the country's vulnerable populations. It's a single-dose shot, meaning it would be suitable for people who found it difficult to travel to vaccination centers—and, unlike the mRNA vaccines, it could be stored at normal refrigerator temperatures. The vaccine also had fewer side effects—both Pfizer and Moderna vaccines could bring on flu-like symptoms such as chills and fever, which might have meant missing work or being retested for Covid.

Delivery of the single-dose J&J vaccine was "paused" in the US after a month, however, when six women developed blood clots after receiving the shot. One of the women died. This came shortly after the AstraZeneca vaccine was banned in Denmark for the same reason. However, on April 15, an Oxford study showed that the risk of cerebral venous sinus thrombosis (CVST), or blood clots, was far greater from contracting Covid-19 than it was from receiving the AstraZeneca vaccine. Of 500,000 cases considered in the study, thirty-nine patients per million experienced CVST from Covid-19, whereas only five per million developed blood clots after being vaccinated. According to Maxime Taquet of Oxford's department of psychiatry (Reuters, April 15, 2021), "the risk of having a (CVST) after Covid-19 appears to be substantially and significantly higher than it is after receiving the Oxford-AstraZeneca vaccine."

Still, AstraZeneca remained off the list of approved vaccines in the US. In Ontario, first doses of Astra-Zeneca were halted in early May 2021, when eight people—out of 853,000 doses administered—experienced vaccine-induced immune thrombotic thrombocytopenia (VITT) after receiving the vaccine. The 50,000 doses of AstraZeneca left in the province were given to citizens as their second dose. In the meantime, Ontario's chief medical officer, Dr. David Williams, said the National Advisory Committee on Immunization (NACI) was "providing direction" on giving Pfizer or Moderna as a second dose to those who had received AstraZeneca as a first dose.

In early June, the go-ahead was given to follow first doses of AstraZeneca with second doses of Pfizer or Moderna, as was already being done in most European countries. A study in Spain, reported in *Nature,* found that mixing two brands of vaccines actually gave a more robust boost to the immune system than two doses of the same vaccine. This general advisory was reversed a month later, when international health authorities maintained that the second dose should be of the same vaccine as the first. The CDC declared on December 17, 2021, that "if you received the first dose of a Pfizer-BioNTech or Moderna Covid-19 vaccine, you should get the same product for your 2nd shot."

In countries besides the US, Germany, and Belgium, other labs were producing their own vaccines. Russia, India, China, Switzerland, South Korea, Cuba, Brazil, South Africa, and Iran all released vaccines based on a number of different approaches. By September 2021, more than twenty vaccines had been approved for use around the world, and a dozen more were undergoing clinical trials. Few of those were approved outside their own countries, but those developed in Russia and India were widely distributed.

Russia's Sputnik V is a nonreplicating (or inactivated) viral vector vaccine, which means the virus it contains is genetically modified so that it cannot replicate inside the host cells. The vaccine, produced by Gamaleya, was the first to be registered anywhere in the world, having been approved for emergency use in Russia in August 2020—a month before the results of its Phase I and Phase II trials were announced. Subsequent trials suggested it was safe and had an efficacy rating of 91.56 percent. Although the vaccine was subsequently approved in seventy countries, the WHO and the European Medicines Agency (EMA) withheld approval, claiming that the manufacturing process in one of Gamaleya's plants did not meet the WHO's standards.

Novavax, based in Maryland, was one of the pharmaceutical companies hailed by Donald Trump in March 2020 as the most likely to produce a Covid vaccine in the shortest time. Trump backed his confidence with an award estimated to be between $1.6 and $1.75 billion, but the Novavax vaccine didn't go to clinical trials until February 2021. Finally, in November 2021, Novavax applied for authorization in the EU, Australia, Canada, the Philippines, and the UK, but its vaccine has not been approved in the US.

Called NVX-CoV2373, the vaccine works differently from others in that it is a "protein subunit vaccine," which means it uses a fragment of a coronavirus spike protein to dupe the human cell into launching an immune-system response. The company claimed it is 89.4 percent effective against the Alpha variant, but it slipped to 49.4 percent against the Beta variant. A large trial conducted in December 2021 found that it was 90 percent effective against the Delta variant, and in December 2021, Reuters reported that the Novavax vaccine was one-quarter as effective against the Omicron variant as it had been against the original coronavirus, but that a third shot of Novavax induced a 73.5-fold increase in antibody levels against Omicron, as opposed to a 25-fold boost by Pfizer and a 37-fold boost by Moderna.

The best-known vaccine produced in India is Covishield, which is the Oxford-AstraZeneca vaccine manufactured under license by the Serum Institute of India. A second vaccine, produced by Bharat Biotech in India, called Covaxin (or BBV152), was approved for emergency use in that country in January 2021, although Phase III trials had not been completed. Phase II trials, which began in June 2020, showed that Covaxin was 62.6 percent effective in asymptomatic patients, 77.8 percent effective in symptomatic patients, and 65.2 percent effective in patients with the Delta variant (the variant that first showed up in India). The vaccine was subsequently approved for emergency use in ten countries in Africa and South America.

The speed at which Covid-19 vaccines were made available was partly because Western scientists were already working on coronavirus vaccines and lipid-based delivery platforms, but also because developed nations could afford the high cost of development. According to *The Lancet*, in 2018 the investment for developing a typical vaccine and launching clinical trials was between $31 and $68 million. When the pandemic hit, poorer countries couldn't afford such a huge outlay, and even wealthy countries in Europe and North America went into debt to fund vaccine research. The European Commission pledged $8 billion to assist in rapid vaccine development. In the US, Operation Warp Speed partnered with the National Institutes of Health and the CDC to come up with $600 million to help pharmaceutical companies produce a vaccine. In the UK, in addition to the 100 million doses it had already ordered from AstraZeneca, the Vaccine Taskforce in July 2020 preordered (and prepaid for) 30 million doses of the Pfizer vaccine and 60 million doses of a vaccine called Valneva being developed in France and Austria (this order was later canceled).

Profits from the sale of vaccines have been astronomical. Some companies, like AstraZeneca and Johnson & Johnson, initially made their vaccines available on a nonprofit basis. Moderna, whose only commercial product is its Covid vaccine, and which lost $514 million in 2019, opted to sell its product for profit; the company disclosed a revenue of $4.4 billion in the three months ending in June 2021 and projected sales of $18.4 billion for the year. Pfizer, having declined government aid in developing its vaccine, elected to sell it for profit and reported $9.2 billion in sales in the second quarter of 2021, compared with $1.2 billion during the same quarter of 2020. According to *Forbes*, Pfizer projects a revenue of $33.5 billion from vaccine sales in 2021.

Rollout / *The process by which Covid-19 vaccines were made available to the public.*

Although it sounds military, the term "rollout" originally referred to the rolling out of a red carpet for the pope. In 1947, however, it was skyjacked by the aeronautics industry to refer to the time in which an aircraft rolls along a runway between landing and coming to a complete stop. More recently, it has referred to the unveiling of a new aircraft: when an airplane or spacecraft prototype is literally rolled out of the hangar for public viewing. In all of its meanings, a rollout has had as much to do with publicity as it has with motion.

"Vaccine rollout across the country," noted Canada's CTV News on February 15, 2021, "has been off to a rocky and slow start." Shortages of vaccines in December 2020 arose when the two companies with which Health Canada had contracts—Pfizer-BioNTech and Moderna—sent only a small percentage of the agreed-upon doses, claiming difficulties with production. The doses that were received were rolled out to the provinces and, within each province, distributed according to vulnerability and the severity of the pandemic in a given region, with health-care workers, the elderly, and the immunocompromised at the front of the line.

By July 30, 2021, 68 million doses of three vaccines—Canada had approved a third vaccine, AstraZeneca, for citizens older than eighteen—had been administered across Canada, and 42.7 percent of the population had been fully vaccinated—at the time defined as having had two doses. In the US, 48 percent of the population had received second doses. Although these figures varied in different parts of both countries, and the average was far short of the herd immunity threshold of 70–80 percent, it meant that the virus's reproduction number was below 1 in some places. In Ontario, the R_0 was 0.84; in all of Canada, only Nova Scotia, at 0.33, and Nunavut, at 0.015, were lower. With the coming of the Omicron variant in December 2021, those R_0 figures went way up.

Elsewhere in the world, the figures were startling. In August 2021, the *Journal of Travel Medicine* published a survey of more than 13,000 studies that had calculated Delta's R_o and found that it ranged from 3.2 to as high as 8, with a mean value of 5.08.

Despite such high reproduction numbers, Canada began easing international travel restrictions; by July 2021, fully vaccinated Canadians and permanent residents returning to Canada were allowed to skip the fourteen-day quarantine period, although they still had to show the results of a negative PCR test that was fewer than three days old. The ban on discretionary travel between Canada and the US by fully vaccinated travelers was lifted on August 9.

In June 2021, BBC News ran the headline "What's Gone Wrong With Australia's Vaccine Rollout?" Although early lockdowns, stay-at-home regulations, and border closings had kept Covid-19 from spreading throughout the country—by then "fortress Australia," with a population of over 25 million, had had 30,274 cases and 910 deaths—only about 3 percent of the population and only 2 percent of people living in long-term care facilities had been fully vaccinated, after vaccines had been available for five months. A shortage of supplies was blamed in part. Most of Australia's doses were AstraZeneca, and after that company failed to meet its obligations within the European Union in March, Italy held back 250,000 doses meant for Australia, which then ordered 40 million doses of the

Pfizer vaccine, expecting to receive them at the rate of 2 million doses a week. However, the first shipment of 457,000 doses didn't arrive until September 2021, a week before the country expanded its rollout to include twelve- to fifteen-year-olds.

China, with its population of 1.4 billion spread out over an area the size of Canada, faced enormous rollout challenges. Distribution of China's vaccines began slowly, with only 100 million doses administered during April 2021. The government vowed that 40 percent of the country would be fully vaxxed by the end of June, meaning the rollout had to be increased fourfold. And it was: in June, 100 million doses a week were administered, and on June 21, China's National Health Commission (NHC) announced that 1.2 billion doses had been administered.

Not all of them were second doses, however, and so the rollout was increased again. By the end of August, 76 percent of the population had received at least one dose, and 889.4 million were fully vaccinated. However, the efficacy of Chinese vaccines was relatively low. "The efficacy of Chinese vaccines is about 70 percent," said China's top respirologist, Zhong Nanshan, citing a figure that may have been optimistic, "so the country would need more than 80 percent of the population to be vaccinated before establishing herd immunity."

Rollouts became more complex when the Delta variant began sweeping through China, and the NHC determined that a third shot was needed to protect even the fully vaccinated from the disease. These booster shots were given to people with compromised immune systems, seniors over sixty years of age, airport staff who were most exposed to imported cases, and those who had to travel abroad, such as airline personnel and foreign students. By the end of 2021, 1.2 billion of China's 1.4 billion people had been fully vaccinated, an extraordinary achievement. But despite the success of its rollout policies, China—like every other country in the world—was still a long way from herd immunity. In January 2022, an average of only 57.9 percent of the world population had received at least one dose of a vaccine, and in poorer countries, that figure was 9.5 percent.

Vaccine Diplomacy / *The practice of one country sending doses of Covid-19 vaccine to another to improve its diplomatic relationship with, or to procure favors from, that country. Also the practice of withholding vaccine doses from another country to punish it for perceived acts of aggression.*

Early in 2021, Russia exported significant quantities of Sputnik V, its homegrown Covid-19 vaccine, to Hungary and Serbia, even though Sputnik V had not been approved by the European Medicines Agency (EMA). The move was seen by some as an attempt to sow discord between EU member countries that abided by EU regulations and those that looked outside the EU for relief, succumbing to the threat of another Covid outbreak. In March, a shipment of 200,000 Sputnik V doses went to Slovakia at the request of Slovakian prime minister Igor Matovič. Following protests against the purchase, Matovič resigned from office. Both France and Germany considered ordering Sputnik V, despite a warning from the EMA that the vaccine had not been properly tested in European labs. In Argentina, President Alberto Fernández tested positive for Covid-19 after having received two doses of Sputnik V.

The very name of the vaccine seems a provocative reference to the Soviet Union's victory in the race for space flight during the Cold War. Now the offer of a Russian vaccine was seen as another of Russia's attempts to destabilize the political systems of other countries—as when Russian hackers allegedly influenced the outcome of the 2016 US elections and continued to distribute fake news to white supremacists and anti-vaxxers. As one BBC News reporter put it, "Russia normally has to spend huge amounts of money on computer hacking and disinformation to spread discord and uncertainty in Europe. Now the vaccine appears to be achieving something similar without any effort."

That has certainly been the case in Ukraine. In early February 2021, according to the website Politico, Russia sent thousands of doses of Sputnik V to rebel-held areas in the country which, with support from Moscow, had been trying to break away from the

Ukraine government in Kyiv since 2004. In December, Russia instituted a mass vaccination drive in the Crimean Peninsula, which Moscow had annexed in 2014, despite protests from Kyiv that the Sputnik V vaccine had not been approved in the EU. "These developments come," reported Politico, "as Sputnik's global rollout is attracting more attention, including from the European Commission, over Moscow's geopolitical motives." Putin used doses of Sputnik V to pave the way for his invasion of Ukraine in February 2022.

In February 2021, The Conversation reported that Israel had agreed to pay Russia to send doses of Sputnik V to Syria as part of a prisoner exchange arrangement. Also that month, China sent half a million doses of its Sinopharm vaccine to Pakistan as a "manifestation of our brotherhood." In March, in a gesture of vaccine diplomacy, the United States exported 2.5 million doses of AstraZeneca vaccine to Mexico and 1.5 million to Canada, marking the first time the US had exported vaccine to another country.

"The prospect of global health becoming a new arena for global power competition and rivalry should worry us all," writes Michael Jennings on The Conversation. The potential fallout would go beyond attempts to create disharmony among rival nations; trading vaccines for political favors or trade deals is a concept that would have had the late John le Carré sharpening his pencils.

The potential to employ vaccine diplomacy within a single country was realized in India, where, as

Arundhati Roy wrote in the *Guardian Weekly* (May 7, 2021), Prime Minister Narendra Modi, campaigning for his party, BJP, in the state of West Bengal, promised voters that if BJP won, "it would ensure people got free vaccines." BJP lost in that state, and the free vaccines failed to appear.

Elaine Dewar, in *On the Origin of the Deadliest Pandemic in 100 Years*, her investigation of the controversial theory that the coronavirus responsible for the Covid-19 pandemic was manufactured in a laboratory in Wuhan, China (see "Lab-Leak Theory"), points to a curious case of vaccine diplomacy involving China and Canada. From 1996 to 2009, Chinese researcher Yu Xuefeng worked for the Canadian branch of the pharmaceutical company Sanofi. In 2009, Yu returned to China and started his own company, CanSino Biologics, where he developed an Ebola vaccine based on a cell line originally crafted in Canada by Dr. Frank Graham. Canada's National Research Council (NRC) had licensed Graham's cell line to CanSino, and another Chinese virologist, Chen Wei, used it to produce Convidecia, China's first Covid-19 vaccine.

"Canada was supposed to have gotten access to that SARS-COV-2 vaccine for phase 1 trials," writes Dewar, "along with the right to manufacture it at an NRC plant being adapted for vaccine production." Then, suddenly, China reneged on the deal, refusing to send any of the vaccine to the NRC. Canada announced that the plan was scrapped because of construction problems at the Montreal plant, but the more likely reason, writes Dewar, lies in the strained relations between Canada and China following the arrest in Vancouver of Huawei CFO Meng Wanzhou, in December 2018, at the request of the American government. The arrest in China of two Canadians, Michael Kovrig and Michael Spavor, was widely seen as an attempt to put pressure on the Canadian government to release Meng Wanzhou; withholding the Covid vaccine is equally obviously another example of the same ploy, "adding," writes Dewar, "vaccine diplomacy to hostage diplomacy in China's bag of pressure tactics."

When Meng Wanzhou was released by Canada in September 2021, the two Michaels were released in China. It's yet to be seen if China will also allow the CanSino vaccine to be produced in Canada. Dr. Scott Halperin, director of the Canadian Center for Vaccinology in Halifax, who had been asked to set up the clinical trials for the CanSino vaccine in Canada, told the CBC in October 2021 that "that vaccine will likely never come to Canada at this stage. It's going to be used around the world in other places, but not in Canada."

Vaccine Nationalism / *The practice of one country accumulating and hoarding vaccine doses rather than sharing them with countries that remain undervaccinated.*

The phrase "vaccine nationalism" was used by Pakistani novelist and activist Fatima Bhutto in an opinion piece published in the *Guardian Weekly* on March 17, 2021. She may have been responding to a statement of newly elected US president Joe Biden, who had said earlier that month that he intended "to start off making sure Americans are taken care of first" before he would consider exporting vaccine doses to other countries. "This petty vaccine nationalism," writes Bhutto, "is irreparably damaging the West, betraying their claims to magnanimity, inclusive global leadership and concern for global health."

Bhutto pointed out that the West, with only 18 percent of the world's population, had acquired 87 percent of the global supply of vaccine doses, a situation she called "morally indefensible." As *New York Times* correspondent Spencer Bokat-Lindell also noted, although there was enough vaccine to inoculate 80 percent of the world's population, in some counties fewer than one person in four would receive a dose. While some wealthy nations had accumulated as many as twenty doses per capita, Bhutto reckoned that "nine out of ten people in poor countries may never be vaccinated at all."

In 2021, Russia and China exported 800 million doses of vaccines developed in their countries to forty-one countries that couldn't afford the Pfizer or Moderna vaccines, whereas the European Union sent out only 34 million doses and the US a mere 4 million—to Canada and Mexico, and only then because the US had huge stockpiles of the AstraZeneca vaccine that were close to their expiration date—and the US Department of Health and Human Services hadn't approved Astra-Zeneca for use in that country.

Vaccine nationalism is a nearsighted strategy even if the goal is to safeguard the health of Western nations. The WHO has said that for the pandemic to be defeated anywhere, it has to be defeated everywhere. If SARS-COV-2 remains rampant in the developing world, it or a deadlier variant of it will eventually return to the developed world to wreak renewed havoc there—as has already happened. Also, economists calculate that developing nations unable to produce goods needed by Western manufacturers because of Covid could cost the global economy $9 trillion.

UN secretary-general António Guterres noted that the world was on the brink of "a catastrophic moral failure." Fatima Bhutto believes the world is long past that brink. "It was the hyper-capitalists who spread the plague," she writes in the *Guardian Weekly* article cited above, "got rich off the vaccine, and now will heal comfortably, first in the queue for the best vaccines that they don't even want. The poor who struggled to eat and survive, lockdown after lockdown, will wait in line and die."

Vaccine Apartheid / *"A situation in which the populations of advanced, rich countries are safely inoculated,"* said South African president Cyril Ramaphosa on May 10, 2021, *"while millions in poorer countries die in the queue would be tantamount to vaccine apartheid."*

Ramaphosa was using a phrase coined earlier by Asia Russell, executive director of Health GAP, an organization that had been advocating, for over two decades, for equal access to medicine around the world, especially for people with HIV. Russell wasn't just calling for a more equitable distribution of vaccines; she was calling for nothing less than a reform of the world's intellectual property laws. "Pharmaceutical companies must wake up," she told openDemocracy on February 26, 2021. "Donation schemes and feel-good initiatives won't fix vaccine apartheid. They must relinquish their patents, share their know-how, and co-operate."

In May 2021, UNICEF estimated poor countries needed 140 million vaccine doses immediately, and WHO director-general Tedros Adhanom Ghebreyesus encouraged specific pharmaceutical companies in wealthy countries to make up that shortfall. He asked Pfizer to donate 40 million doses to COVAX, the vaccine-sharing agency started by the WHO, and he urged Moderna to make the doses it had promised for 2022 available in 2021. Speaking at the Paris Peace Forum,

Ghebreyesus noted that COVAX had shipped 63 million doses to 124 countries—but that covered just 0.5 percent of the combined populations of those countries. He called for more sharing of doses but, echoing Russell, also stressed the need for pharmaceutical companies to share their technologies to increase the manufacturing of vaccines worldwide. Referring to the danger of splitting the world into have and have-not nations, Ghebreyesus said, "I think I would go one step further and say not just that the world is at risk of vaccine apartheid; the world is in vaccine apartheid."

By the fall of 2021, still only 0.8 percent of the population of Africa had been fully vaccinated; the figure in the US was 55 percent; in Germany, it was 64 percent; and in Canada, 71 percent. "Rich nations," reported the *New York Times* on July 16, "have bought up most doses long into the future, often far more than they could conceivably need. Hundreds of millions of shots from a global vaccine-sharing effort have failed to materialize." The goal in African countries to have 20 percent fully vaccinated by the end of 2021 "seems out of reach."

The pandemic presented the world's wealthy countries with an opportunity to show compassion for their less fortunate, or less rapacious, neighbors. To put people ahead of profits, and altruism above self-interest. The world's wealthy nations have spectacularly failed the test.

4

The Flight From Science and Reason

"Science has in some quarters come to be looked on as an enemy... I would go so far as to say that the lack of a common frame of reference, the absence of any unifying set of concepts and principles, is now, if not the world's major disease, at least its most serious symptom."

JULIAN HUXLEY, *New Bottles for New Wine*, 1957

"Without science, democracy has no future."

MAXIM GORKY, 1917

Anti-Masker; Anti-Vaxxer /

"That aunt... had judged [Jackson's] fearlessness to be infantile and foolish... 'If his bed was on fire, he'd rather sleep with flames than run for water. Like a fool. If there was plague in the house, he'd rather die than cover his nose.'" JIM CRACE, *The Pesthouse*

A person strongly opposed to wearing a face mask or being vaccinated during the Covid-19 pandemic. Not always, but often, the same person.

The term "anti-masker" appeared on social media in early 2020 to refer to anyone who, despite urgings from family, friends, health professionals, and especially governments, refused to wear a face mask. The epithet was inspired by the term "anti-vaxxer," which was a person who refused to allow their children to be vaccinated, especially against measles, mumps, and rubella (MMR). This earlier anti-vax movement arose following the 1998 publication in *The Lancet* of an article by British virologist Andrew Wakefield, who purported to have linked the MMR vaccine to an increased risk of autism in children.

The connection between vaccines and autism was quickly debunked by epidemiologists around the world. But in 2007, model and actress Jenny McCarthy gave it new life in her book *Louder Than Words: A Mother's Journey in Healing Autism*, and later on *The Oprah Winfrey Show*, where she opined that the MMR vaccine triggered autism. Suddenly, thousands of parents who had never heard of *The Lancet* stopped allowing their children to be vaccinated, and as a result, a disease that had been all but eradicated began a slow but deadly comeback. In 2018, *Nature* referred to a measles epidemic in the Democratic Republic of the Congo that killed 6,000 people as "the largest documented measles outbreak in one country since the world gained a measles vaccine in 1963." That year, worldwide, 140,000 people died of measles, most of them children. But resistance to measles vaccinations persisted, and when the Covid pandemic arrived, it morphed into resistance to Covid vaccines.

There are degrees of anti-vaxxers. The lazy and indifferent—people who can shrug off a disease that has killed at least 15 million people as something that doesn't really affect them—are at one end of the continuum. Most of these eventually become vaccinated, though grudgingly, when their bosses threaten to fire them if they don't. Then there are those who are not anti-vax per se but who are not convinced that getting a vaccine is an effective way to stop the spread of the coronavirus. They have decided to wait and see. These are referred to by the WHO as the "vaccine hesitant"; though not placard-carrying fist-shakers, they nonetheless constitute one of the biggest roadblocks to reducing the spread of Covid. In 2020, the WHO named vaccine hesitancy one of the top ten threats to human health.

True, diehard anti-vaxxers are against vaccination on principle. For either ideological or religious reasons, they believe that the urging of the government to become vaccinated is a plot to undermine their way of life. In January 2022, the website sorryantivaxxer. com, which posts accounts of people who resist being vaccinated, posted the story of a forty-two-year-old man from Virginia who had stage-5 kidney disease and had been removed from a wait list for a kidney transplant because he refused to be vaccinated. "Nobody can tell me with 100 percent certainty," he declares in a YouTube video, "that I will have no adverse reaction" if he gets vaccinated. Even though, as sorryantivaxxer comments, his doctors have told him with 100 percent certainty that he will die if he doesn't.

The CDC has estimated that unvaccinated Covid patients are eleven times as likely as those who have been vaccinated to die of Covid. Dr. Tasleem Nimjee, a Covid-19 task force member at Humber River Hospital in Toronto, told the *Toronto Star* in September 2021 that she often hears patients in her care trying to explain why they aren't vaccinated. "The main themes I hear," she says, "are: 'I don't trust the vaccine'; 'I wanted to wait until a lot of people have the vaccine to help me feel safer'; 'I haven't gotten Covid so far, so I don't think I'm going to get it.'" Dr. Jane Healey, a pediatrician and physician lead for the Trillium Health Partners testing lab in Mississauga, Ontario, has had to tell many unvaccinated patients that their Covid tests were positive. "Sometimes," she says, "they ask if they can have the vaccine now."

Many people also seem to think they're following health guidelines if they keep a face mask in their pocket or pull it down under their nose, or even their chin. When Canadian author Bill Richardson was working in a grocery store in Vancouver at the beginning of the pandemic, part of his job was to offer a free face mask to each incoming customer—at the time, as a convenience, not yet a requirement. About half the customers declined the offer, he writes in his story

"Loss Prevention." The list of excuses people made for not taking a mask is varied and instructive:

I don't need one; I've just had my hair done.

I don't need one; I'm buying vegan ice cream.

I don't need one; I had it back in November when no one knew what it was.

I don't need one; I know a lot of people, none of them is sick, no one is even coughing.

I don't need one; I've got the herd immunity.

None of the customers told him that face masks were part of a government sterilization plot or that mandating mask-wearing denied their right to make other people sick. Many didn't even know themselves why they weren't wearing a mask; they just weren't.

True anti-maskers and anti-vaxxers know exactly why they aren't wearing a mask or getting vaccinated: for the most part, they simply object to being told what to do. They maintain they are not so much anti-mask or anti-vax as anti-mandate or anti-government. In Germany, neologisms used by anti-vaxxers include *Corona-Diktatur*, corona dictatorship, meaning a government that would mandate an *Impfzwang*—forced vaccination. In Berlin, in November 2020, nearly 10,000 anti-maskers demonstrated against mandated restrictions and lockdowns. Some carried posters promoting QAnon; others wore Trump hats emblazoned with "MAGA."

Some demonstrators claimed they did not trust their government to make an intelligent choice when approving an eventual vaccine; others denied that a pandemic existed, insisting that it had been invented by politicians who wanted to sow fear and panic in order to "control the masses," as one demonstrator told the television channel France 24, "as in Hitler's time." That and other anti-mandate demonstrations were organized by a group from Stuttgart called *Querdenken* (lateral thinking), a reference to Edward de Bono's 1967 book *The Use of Lateral Thinking*. Lateral thinkers, said de Bono, think outside the box. They think creatively rather than along the usual well-trodden lines. One of the methods to generate new ways of thinking, de Bono proposed, was to make a statement that we know is wrong.

In an article appearing in *Mother Jones* on January 10, 2018, Megan Jula notes that the popularity of both Oprah Winfrey and Donald Trump provided large and unregulated public platforms for people with unsubstantiated opinions and scarce scientific evidence to reach huge audiences. Jenny McCarthy's views on measles vaccinations would have faded into obscurity had they not been trumpeted by Oprah Winfrey to her 15 million daily viewers. By voicing their own unfounded opinions, so-called "influencers" give tacit permission to others to make similarly unfounded claims. "Trump voters become more anti-vax after reading his tweets," concludes University of Queensland professor Matthew J. Hornsey in the *Journal of Experimental Social Psychology* (May 2020).

"Trump doesn't just *reflect* the views of his supporters, he still has the power to *shape* his supporters' views."

Republican senator Rand Paul publicly stated that vaccines could cause "mental disorders." Refusing to be vaccinated, he said, was "an issue of freedom." Anti-maskers similarly claimed that the decision not to wear a face mask was political, an issue of personal freedom. Anti-mask posters appearing in Toronto proclaimed that "The Mask is a Muzzle" and that being mandated to wear a face mask during a pandemic infringed on their human rights.

In the online magazine Fair Observer (a media partner of the Centre for Analysis of the Radical Right) in November 2020, Bàrbara Molas noted that "conspiracy theories and claims to freedom of choice have characterized the radical-right fight against mandatory mask policies in Canada." According to Molas, 90 percent of Canadians who identify as left-leaning were likely to wear face masks, compared to only 60 percent of those identifying as right-leaning. Right-leaners were also much more likely to link mask-wearing with conspiracy theories such as those promoted by QAnon, which tells followers that a secret cabal of Satan worshippers, including many Democratic senators, is running a child sex-trafficking ring.

Another conspiracy theory holds that vaccines contain microchips that will allow governments to control the mind of anyone who receives a vaccination. Vladislav Sobolev, cofounder of the anti-mask movement

Hugs Over Masks, echoed Rand Paul by maintaining that wearing face masks was dangerous to health and that being forced to wear one was a violation of citizens' freedom. Like the *Querdenken* protesters in Berlin, Sobolev linked "what is happening in Canada [with] the uprising of Nazi Germany," as if requiring all citizens to wear face masks during a pandemic was the same as rounding up specific groups and sending them to death camps.

Can it be a coincidence that after two years of the pandemic, the three countries with the highest per capita death toll due to Covid-19—the United States, Brazil, and the UK—were all led by anti-maskers? In Brazil, President Jair Bolsonaro told a news conference in February 2021, when his country's death toll from Covid was more than 1,500 a day, that wearing a face mask was bad for children because it made concentration difficult and could produce "a decreased perception of happiness." By March 2022, the death rate from Covid in Brazil was the highest in the world: 3,095 per million population. UK prime minister Boris Johnson publicly announced that he had shaken hands with everyone when he visited a coronavirus ward in May 2020. In the United States, Trump's repeated denials of the efficacy of face masks, and his mockery of those who wore them, was seen as a significant factor in that country's high death rate. In October 2020, CDC epidemiologist Robert Hahn charted pandemic-related deaths from April 2020, when Trump declared that wearing masks was "voluntary," to the end of July 2020, when Trump finally admitted that he would wear a mask, and estimated that as many as 12,000 deaths could be attributed to Trump's negative and false assertions about face masks.

A Pew Research Center poll conducted in August 2021 found that the division between those who were vaccinated and those who weren't fell along party lines: 86 percent of Democrats had had at least one dose, whereas only 60 percent of Republicans had. David Leonhardt, writing in the *New York Times* in September 2021, noted that such a sharp partisan division did not exist in other countries: people were pro- or anti-vaccination for various reasons, but not necessarily ideological ones. "What distinguishes the US," he writes, "is a conservative party—the Republican Party—that has grown hostile to science and empirical evidence in recent decades." That month, when the majority of those hospitalized with Covid were unvaccinated, the imbalance in vaccination rates between red Republican and blue Democrat states inspired some to refer to the pandemic as "red Covid."

The US wasn't the only country to have a strong lobby of anti-vaxxers, and usually the difference in death rates was about the same. In November 2021, at the peak of the Omicron wave—when the US recorded 11.9 deaths per 100,000 citizens among unvaccinated patients, compared to 1.12 per 100,000 among the vaccinated—Switzerland had 6.26 deaths per 100,000 among the unvaxxed, and 0.53 among the vaxxed. In Chile, it was 4.87 per 100,000 unvaccinated patients, compared to 1.26 among the vaxxed.

There is a strong correlation between anti-vaxxers and the religious right. In an article in a Texas A&M University liberal arts publication that appeared in May 2021, titled "Why Evangelicals Are Encouraging the Anti-Vaccination Movement," Mia Mercer suggests that evangelicals' belief in the literal interpretation of the Bible and the sovereignty of God makes them reject medical treatment for diseases. "If you get sick," religious studies professor Heidi Campbell told her, "it's because you don't have faith in God and that you're not living a holy life." Receiving a vaccine meant you lacked faith. Mercer cites an example from Uganda, where a hospital received 5,000 doses of a vaccine "but was only able to administer about 400 doses because of vaccine hesitancy among a heavily evangelical population."

Whatever their reasoning, when health authorities began rolling out vaccines, anti-vaxxers played a significant role in ensuring that Covid-19 remained in the population and that people continued to die from it. In June 2021, CDC figures showed that of the 107,000 people hospitalized with Covid in May, only 1,200 of them had been vaccinated. And of the 18,000 deaths that resulted from those hospitalizations, only 150 were of people who had been vaccinated. According to those figures, anti-vaxxers are mainly killing each other.

It may be that anti-vaxxers are simply engaging in "vice signaling," which Noah Berlatsky defines in *The Independent* as "a public display of immorality, intended to create a community based on cruelty and disregard for others, which is proud of it at the same time."

A community is supposed to be based on mutual concern for others; a community based on disregard for others sounds like a hydroxymoron.

Vaccine Hunters / *People so keen to be vaccinated that they wait at a vaccination center or hospital for a vaccine dose, even if they were not scheduled to receive one. The opposite of anti-vaxxers.*

The practice of hunting vaccine doses arose in January 2021, when vaccination centers opened in the US and certain groups of people—such as frontline and health-care personnel, residents of long-term care facilities, people with high-risk health conditions, and the elderly—were scheduled to receive vaccinations before the general population. Those groups were able to register for vaccines online or by telephone, and everyone else was told to wait until the vulnerable and the exposed had been vaccinated. A lot of people didn't want to wait.

The two vaccines approved in the US, those from Pfizer and Moderna, had short shelf lives after being removed from refrigeration—Moderna's was twelve hours and Pfizer's was only two, and after that, the vaccines would have to be either used or destroyed. In the morning, a vaccination center took enough doses out of the freezer for that day's registered recipients, and any doses left unused at the end of the day would have to be discarded. Instead of wasting vaccine, many facilities gave the day's leftover doses to anyone who wanted one. "Vaccine hunters" lined up outside the facilities, "in the often-futile hope of getting a shot," reported the *New York Times*.

Very soon, websites and social media accounts were set up in major cities in the US and Canada that provided up-to-the-minute lists of facilities that were handing out vaccine doses, and also helped people make appointments. VaccineHunter.org in the US inspired Vaccine Hunters Canada, formed in March 2021 "to connect eligible Canadians with vaccination appointments" and to help them navigate their way through government online platforms. In both countries, hundreds of volunteers monitored posts on Twitter, Instagram, TikTok, and other sites to ensure that as many people received vaccines as possible. On September 3, 2021, when most Canadians were vaccinated and the rollouts were running smoothly, Vaccine Hunters Canada wound down. The site's founder,

Andrew Young, estimated that his group had helped 1.2 million Canadians receive vaccinations.

Patent Waiver / *The voluntary relinquishing of Covid vaccine patents belonging to pharmaceutical companies to allow laboratories in low- and middle-income countries to manufacture the vaccines for themselves.*

In February 2020, when the rapidity and extent of the spread of Covid-19 was becoming clear, the World Health Organization held a meeting of public health agencies to work out an "R&D blueprint" for contending with the impending global emergency. One of the steps the group discussed was to facilitate open communication among researchers in rival institutions and in different countries so that efforts weren't wasted and breakthroughs benefited the global community. The WHO and its member organizations assumed that pharmaceutical companies would not allow concerns about intellectual property rights to outweigh the need to protect as much of the world's population as possible. They assumed that corporate executives, and their lawyers and shareholders, would not place profits above people's lives.

For a while, it looked as though that would happen. Alexander Zaitchik, writing in the *New Republic* in April 2021, recalls that planners within the WHO and its implementing partners believed that "public and private actors would collect research and associated intellectual property in a global knowledge fund for the duration of the pandemic." This belief led to the formation of the WHO's COVID-19 Technology Access Pool (C-TAP), which invited all holders of technology-related knowledge to work together so that "shared knowledge, intellectual property and data will leverage our collective efforts to advance scientific discovery, technology development and broad sharing of the benefits of scientific advancement and its applications based on the right to health."

That kind of cooperation for the common good within a free-market, capitalist society, especially when it concerned human health, had had encouraging precedents. In 1922, for example, the year Frederick Banting and Charles Best determined that diabetes was caused by the body's failure to produce insulin, the University of Toronto licensed the Eli Lilly company of Indiana to manufacture and sell insulin in the United States and Central and South America, but kept the rest of the world rights in Canada. In the 1930s, the university was thus able to allow Danish physician H. C. Hagedorn to produce insulin in Scandinavia. At the time, insulin from Eli Lilly had to be injected several times a day to be effective. Hagedorn realized that by adding protamine to insulin, a single injection would last up to twenty-four hours.

Hagedorn shared his discovery with Canadian scientists D. A. Scott and A. M. Fisher, who added zinc to insulin to make an injection last up to thirty-six hours. This was a clear case of an open sharing of technology between Canadian and Danish scientists that advanced the cause of human health far beyond what a commercial corporation like Eli Lilly—which obviously made more money if patients needed multiple injections a day—had been able or willing to accomplish.

Working on the principle that we were all in the pandemic together, and that health is a basic human right, C-TAP launched as an "open science" initiative that would make vaccine information available to not-for-profit agencies in lower- and middle-income countries. "The world has an overwhelming interest in ensuring [vaccines] will be universally and cheaply available," lauded the *Financial Times*. C-TAP would "compile, in one place, pledges of commitment made... to voluntarily share Covid-19 health technology, related knowledge, intellectual property and data."

One of the member partners was the Medicines Patent Pool (MPP), which had already been providing researchers in lower- and middle-income countries with open access to advances in treatment for HIV, hepatitis C, and tuberculosis. Another was Tech Access Partnership (TAP), a United Nations organization created to "facilitate connections between experienced manufacturers and local manufacturers in developing countries to share key data, knowledge and other relevant support through a coordinated network."

Standing in the way of this altruistic initiative, however, was the Agreement on Trade-Related Aspects of Intellectual Property Rights (TRIPS), signed in 1994 by all members of the World Trade Organization (WTO). According to TRIPS, each signatory nation would recognize and respect the intellectual property rights of the other member nations. In October 2020, however, the leaders of India and South Africa (two countries hard-hit by extremely high rates of Covid-19 infections and deaths, and short on the prospect of vaccines) petitioned the WTO to issue a waiver on the TRIPS agreement—in other words, to allow companies in their countries to manufacture Covid vaccines rather than wait for premanufactured doses to be shipped from the US and Europe. South Africa and India were, in effect, asking the WTO to honor an international agreement signed seven years after TRIPS—the Doha Declaration of 2001—which stated that, in times of emergency, TRIPS could and should be waived in favor of the goal "to promote access to medicines for all." South Africa, India, and the hundred other countries that joined them in petitioning the WTO, as David Adler and Mamka Anyona put it in the *Guardian Weekly* (May 7, 2021), "knew then what has become apparent to everyone now: the system of pharmaceutical patents is a killing machine."

As the WTO and several first world countries considered the proposal, Bill Gates entered the discussion. A billionaire businessman for whom the idea of a corporation relinquishing patented information so that another company could manufacture its product was anathema, he felt that companies that had devoted billions of dollars and a great deal of energy to developing vaccines against Covid-19 should be allowed to profit from their efforts. Otherwise, he stated, why would they bother? "It's the classic situation in global health," he told the CBC in January 2021. "The advocates all of a sudden want it for zero dollars and right away. And I feel these pharma companies that jumped in, well... they're the reason we can see the end of the epidemic coming."

If Gates could see the end of the "epidemic" in January 2021, he had greater foresight than the world's top health professionals. But his business philosophy gelled with that of most politicians in the West. His solution to the problem of vaccine shortages was to ensure that lower- and middle-income countries received enough vaccine doses to immunize the same proportion of their population as in rich countries. Pharmaceutical companies in the US, for example, could make the vaccines and sell them, at a sliding scale from full price to at cost, to poor countries. Through the Bill & Melinda Gates Foundation, GAVI (the Global Alliance for Vaccines and Immunization, later called Gavi, the Vaccine Alliance), and the WHO, Gates committed billions of dollars to COVAX, the WHO's international initiative to distribute vaccines more equitably to low- and middle-income countries. Rather than share the formulas so that poorer countries could manufacture their own vaccines, COVAX purchased vaccine doses from pharmaceutical companies and distributed them to countries that were lagging behind in vaccination rates. Gates and COVAX committed to delivering 2.3 billion doses of vaccines by the end of 2021, 1.8 billion of which would go to poor countries "at no cost" to the countries themselves.

This announcement took much of the wind out of patent waiver's sails. Since then, wealthy countries have cooled on the idea of relinquishing patented information. The European Union said it was "considering the proposal," but European Commission president Ursula von der Leyen refused to endorse the plan, saying it would be better to export vaccines to poorer countries, which was Bill Gates's plan. Germany thought waivers might undermine production, another way of saying that without the profit incentive, pharmaceutical companies would lose interest in manufacturing vaccines that would save millions of lives.

This suggestion, or threat, had also been made during the AIDS pandemic, when pharmaceutical companies balked at allowing poorer countries to make their own antiretroviral drugs. As Gregg Gonsalves, an AIDS activist and epidemiologist at the Yale School of

Public Health, told the *New York Times* in June 2021, "back then, we were also told, 'Don't you dare support other countries making generic antiretroviral drugs or else you are going to destroy the goose that lays the golden egg. You'll never see another AIDS drug again for the rest of your life.' It's completely not true," he said. The WTO waived patents for a number of "least-developed countries" in Africa and Asia, and yet "the pharmaceutical industry has prospered and thrived."

Opposing waivers on another front, a spokesperson for Germany said that "the limiting factor in vaccine manufacturing is production capacity and high-quality standards, not patents," suggesting that low-income countries had neither the capacity nor the expertise to produce their own vaccines. But the idea behind C-TAP had not been simply to send formulas to companies in lower- and middle-income countries, but also to supply the technology and expertise to turn those formulas into vaccines. It was to be a true gift; wealthy countries were not just handing out fish but also supplying the means for poorer countries to catch fish on their own.

COVAX may have ensured that lower- and middle-income countries received more doses than they otherwise would have, but by May 2021 it was clear that equitable distribution was not happening. Moderna's production difficulties made it impossible to fulfill even its domestic commitments. Pfizer continued to make money selling vaccines to rich countries, while in countries like India people continued to die for lack of vaccines and adequate hospital care, especially oxygen, which one would think would be plentiful. As Hannah Ellis-Petersen writes in *The Guardian*, "while India's Covid-19 cases have continued to surge at record-breaking pace, with the country registering 368,147 new cases and a further 3,417 deaths on Monday [May 3], the rate of vaccinations across the country has fallen to its lowest levels." Arundhati Roy writes that, because not everyone in India who became sick was tested or hospitalized, the actual death rate in India was likely to be "up to 30 times higher than the official count."

In the first three months of 2021, while thousands died in India, Africa, and South America, Pfizer earned $3.5 billion from vaccine sales and projected a profit of $14 billion by the end of the year. Although its CEO, Albert Bourla, declared that poor countries "have the same access as the rest of the world" to their product, the WHO's statistics showed otherwise: rich countries had received 87 percent of vaccine doses, while lower- and middle-income received less than 1 percent. Even Bill Gates acknowledged that with COVAX there would be a six- to eight-month gap between rich countries and poor countries receiving sufficient vaccinations to "defeat" Covid.

On May 6, 2021, US president Joe Biden announced his support for waiving intellectual property protections, setting off a barrage of angry responses from pharma companies and organizations. Michelle McMurry-Heath, president and CEO of the Biotechnology Innovation Organization (BIO), was "extremely disappointed" by Biden's "myopic decision," saying that "handing needy countries a recipe book without the ingredients, safeguards, and sizable workforce needed will not help people waiting for the vaccine." Albert Bourla, Pfizer's CEO, sent an open letter to Pfizer employees assuring them that "fair and equitable distribution... was our North Star from day one," but that "the suggested waiver of [intellectual property] rights could only derail this progress." Allowing low- and middle-income countries to manufacture their own vaccines, he said, would set off a scramble for the raw materials needed to make them, threatening every country's ability to make enough vaccine to deal with the pandemic. "Entities with little or no experience in manufacturing vaccines are likely to chase the very raw materials we require to scale our production, putting the safety and security of all at risk." Sending experienced technicians and links to material sources, along with the vaccine formulas, doesn't seem to have occurred to anyone.

Bourla's objection was a red herring, however, since the US controlled the raw materials needed to manufacture vaccines, and those materials were protected by trade agreements that Biden couldn't circumvent. According to *The Guardian* (April 10, 2021), one of the reasons the Serum Institute of India was unable to supply India with enough Covishield was that "the US government has ... blocked exports of [bioreactor] bags, filters, and other components so it can supply more Pfizer vaccines for Americans."

At any rate, Biden quickly backed down on his support for patent waivers. On May 17, he announced that the US would send 20 million doses of Pfizer, Moderna, and J&J vaccines overseas, and told the *New York Times* that, "unlike Russia and China ... the United States will not expect any favors in return." In neither Biden's announcement nor the *Times* article was the phrase "patent waiver" mentioned.

In mid-April, WTO director-general Ngozi Okonjo-Iweala proposed on the WHO's website what she called "a third way" to approach the problem of unequal distribution of vaccines, "in which we can license manufacturing to countries so that you can have adequate supplies while still making sure that intellectual property issues are taken care of." The model Okonjo-Iweala proposed was something like the licensing arrangement by which the Serum Institute of India (SII) was manufacturing the AstraZeneca vaccine under the name Covishield. SII is the biggest manufacturer of vaccines in the world, capable of producing a billion doses of Covishield a month; enough, it said, to vaccinate the entire world by the end of 2022. AstraZeneca still holds the patent on its vaccine, but SII pays the company a fee to manufacture it in India. AstraZeneca has even said it will not profit from sales of

Covishield as long as the pandemic lasts, although, as NPR noted on March 18, 2021, the company added that "it reserves the right to declare a legal end to the pandemic as early as this July." It might even have been able to do so, had more countries been allowed to manufacture their own vaccines.

Vaccine Shedding / *A minor phenomenon of live vaccines mistakenly cited to justify anti-vaxxers' belief that inoculation against Covid-19 gives a person Covid-19.*

In April 2021, the Centner Academy, a private elementary school in Miami, told its teachers that getting vaccinated against Covid-19 would cost them their jobs. Vaccinated teachers would not be allowed into the classrooms. One of the teachers who agreed with the policy warned his fifth-grade students that if they hugged their parents who had been vaccinated, they could contract Covid-19. The reason for this precaution, announced the school's owner, Leila Centner, was her belief in the reality of "vaccine shedding."

Citing vaccine shedding as a threat was a ploy of anti-vaccination groups trying to discourage or intimidate as many people as possible into resisting being vaccinated. Mass emails were sent out warning that coming into contact with "the vaccinated" could cause postmenopausal women to begin menstruating again or pregnant women to miscarry, or that vaccination could result in stillbirths. These groups maintained that being vaccinated caused the body to "shed" the coronavirus's spike proteins, which somehow were transmitted to others and somehow caused ill effects.

Vaccine shedding is a real phenomenon, but it only happens when patients receive a live virus vaccine, and even then the probability of infection through shedding is only 0.58 percent. Very few Covid-19 vaccines are live-virus—almost all of them use either killed or inactivated viruses, attenuated viruses (live viruses that have been genetically altered to replicate without causing illness), or isolated proteins. The mRNA vaccines contain no virus at all, just a genetic instruction. The live virus technique was used in the 1950s with the Salk polio vaccine, and there was some transmission by vaccine shedding then—entirely through stool contamination—but with improved sanitation and almost no use of live virus vaccines, there is virtually no danger of a person vaccinated against Covid endangering anyone who comes into contact with them through vaccine shedding.

According to Zubin Damania—a former Stanford University School of Medicine physician better known as ZDoggMD, an award-winning blogger and YouTuber on health issues—the fear of vaccine shedding lies in the observation that syncytin, a protein involved in placental formation in pregnant women, is structurally similar to the spike protein in coronaviruses. But the fear of vaccine shedding is a falsehood perpetrated by anti-vaxxers for their own political and social agendas. The Centner Academy elementary school charges an annual tuition of $30,000, and since Leila Centner's campaign against vaccination began, it has been contacted by thousands of parents who want to enroll their children. Centner herself, a firm Republican who supported (and still supports) Donald Trump, says she espouses "medical freedom" for the students in her school. But not, apparently, for the teachers.

Waning Immunity / *The gradual decline of antibodies in people who have been fully vaccinated against Covid.*

In July 2021, a paper released by Health Canada found that protection from vaccines administered from December 2020 to July 2021 had dropped from 90 to 40 percent in people aged sixty-five years and older and recommended that third shots be given to that demographic as soon as possible. The report spurred a number of investigations in other countries. In September, a New York State Department of Health study found a "modest decline" in immunity in New Yorkers who had received their second dose between May and August. "The findings of our study," wrote Dr. Eli Rosenberg, the paper's lead author, "support the need for boosters in older people in particular."

The New York study echoed similar surveys conducted in the UK, which found that the AstraZeneca, Moderna, and Pfizer vaccines all declined in effectiveness ten weeks after the second dose. None of the vaccines declined very dramatically, however; Pfizer stated that its effectiveness rating dropped from 96 percent to 84 percent after six months, and Moderna reported effectiveness dropped from 94 percent to a number "greater than 90" in that same time period.

Scientists involved in these studies assured everyone that "we shouldn't worry about a few percentage points," but by then, health officials in half a dozen countries, including the US, the United Arab Emirates, China, Israel, and Russia, had already started worrying. On August 12, the US FDA approved booster shots for some recipients of either the Pfizer or Moderna vaccine, and a week later the US Department of Health and Human Services announced that every American over the age of twelve should get a third shot eight months after having received their second one.

Before Omicron, the response from scientists was that giving widespread third doses was unnecessary, and possibly even counterproductive. Studies suggesting that immunity waned six months after the second dose looked only at the presence of antibodies, but immunity isn't measured solely by antibodies. "Antibodies are *supposed* to peter out," writes Katherine J. Wu in *The Atlantic*. What matters for long-term immunity is the continued presence of memory B cells, and these become stronger as time goes on. At the time of vaccination, the body produces masses of antibodies to ward off the coronavirus, but most of those are ineffective against a specific virus; they just overwhelm the invader without paying too much attention to what kind of invader it is. After a few weeks, they wane, and the memory B cells go into action. These memory cells produce more antibodies, selecting those that specifically seek out coronaviruses, and these new antibodies stick around longer, for up to fifteen weeks. When they eventually fade, the memory B cells remain on guard in the event of a reinfection, in which case they almost instantly produce an armada of specifically evolved antibodies—and if the body becomes infected at all, it's with only a mild version of Covid. Most immunologists agree that, unless a patient has a compromised immune system, a third shot isn't a good idea.

Which is why the who called a moratorium on third-shot discussions in August 2021, asking countries to hold off on booster shots until the end of September, except for those who were immunocompromised. Most first world countries went ahead and scheduled general boosters anyway—the European Union wanted everyone in Europe, whether they had compromised immune systems or not, to be triple-vaxxed. This prompted who director-general Tedros Adhanom Ghebreyesus to comment in October that booster shots for healthy citizens of wealthy countries was "immoral, unfair and unjust, and it has to stop." Africa, said

Ghebreyesus, was still only 7 percent vaccinated, and many people there had not yet had a single vaccination. "To start boosters is really the worst we can do as a global community," he stated. "We will not stop the pandemic by ignoring a whole continent."

Omicron changed all that, however. Early studies in South Africa, where Omicron was first detected, suggested that the new variant lowered the effectiveness of vaccines. One study showed that when the blood of people double-vaccinated with the Pfizer vaccine was exposed to different variants, the antibody response to Omicron showed a forty-one-fold decline compared to earlier variants. UK studies showed similar results after the AstraZeneca vaccine. By mid-December 2021, most wealthy countries had made third shots available to the majority of their citizens; the *British Medical Journal (BMJ)* reported on December 17 that "over 365 million booster or third shots have been administered globally."

Governments embraced boosters largely because they had little else to offer a population faced with a new variant and tired of what Nesrine Malik, in *The Guardian* (December 20, 2021), called "the uncertainty, the stop-starts, that marooned feeling of waiting to be rescued, the anticipation of life changing overnight," which she blamed mainly on government ineptitude. Scientists remained divided on the need for boosters, but generally came down against recommending them. As K. Srinath Reddy writes in *The Lancet* on October 29, 2021, if wealthier countries once again used up the lion's share of vaccine doses, "under-vaccinated populations could generate the conditions for the emergence of new variants." In other words, universal boosterism might help flatten the Omicron curve, but it could also pave the way for an even more virulent and transmissible variant later on.

In early January 2022, booster shots were made available to all US citizens over the age of twelve, six months after they had received their second doses of an mRNA vaccine. According to *Yale Medicine*, boosters can trigger the immune system to begin producing more antibodies immediately, meaning that immunocompromised patients need not just hope that their memory B cells will kick in. Boosters, therefore, "became increasingly important as the highly contagious Omicron variant caused a surge in cases."

5

The Demon of Noontide

"...that which the Greeks call 'a-kedia' and which
we may describe as tedium or perturbation of heart.
It is akin to dejection and especially felt by wandering
monks and solitaries, a persistent and obnoxious
enemy to such as dwell in the desert, disturbing the monk
especially about midday, like a fever mounting at a regular
time, and bringing its highest tide of inflammation at
definite accustomed hours to the sick soul. And so some
of the Fathers declare it to be the demon of noontide
which is spoken of in the [ninety-first] Psalm."

CASSIAN OF MARSEILLES, *Desert Father*, fourth century CE

"Thou shalt not be afraid for the terror by night;
nor for the arrow that flieth by day;
Nor for the pestilence that walketh in darkness;
nor for the destruction that wasteth at noonday."

PSALM 91:5–6

Coronaphobia / *The exaggerated fear of contracting Covid-19.*

In a study published in the *Asian Journal of Psychiatry* in December 2020, Alisha Arora and three coauthors note that in its first year the pandemic had already had "multiple socioeconomic and psychological ramifications," including "a rise in fears related to contracting the virus." This presented "a new emerging phobia specific to Covid-19." People suffering from "coronaphobia," she said, exhibited "excessive concern over physiological symptoms, significant stress about personal and occupational loss, increased reassurance and safety seeking behaviors, and avoidance of public places and situations, causing marked impairment in daily life functioning."

Coronaphobia is classified as a form of obsessive-compulsive disorder. Apparently, compulsive hand-washing is not much different from compulsive hoarding of toilet paper (hoarding coffee I can understand—I've got fifteen bags of Kicking Horse in my cupboard—but toilet paper?). Coronaphobic reactions can be triggered by such factors as unforeseen realities (on-again, off-again restrictions), unending uncertainties (will the schools be open on Monday? what the hell is "Deltacron"?), the need to acquire new practices and avoidance techniques (should I do my grocery shopping at midnight?), and loss of faith in political leaders (if people had much to begin with).

When these reactions begin to interfere with routine life—causing one to misinterpret benign symptoms as signs of illness, for example, or to amplify one's risk of contracting Covid—the person is said to be suffering from a phobia. Coronaphobia is similar to agoraphobia, except that agoraphobia is a fear of open places, whereas coronaphobia is a fear of the people in those places (as well as a fear of people in enclosed spaces).

Physiological symptoms of coronaphobia include a rapid heart rate, trouble breathing, sweating, and sleep disturbances or deprivation. When coronaphobia is triggered by a fear of unforeseen circumstances, as may be experienced during lockdowns, quarantines, and self-isolation, psychiatrists perceive a similarity with a phobia experienced by prisoners: chronophobia, or the fear of time.

"Chronophobia . . . is a common experience for those in quarantine," write Ahmed Naguy et al. in another 2020 paper from the *Asian Journal of Psychiatry*, "a neurotic fear of time typically described in prison neurosis where duration and immensity of time is utterly terrifying to [the] prisoner and passage of time throws him into a panic. At a later stage, people become phlegmatic automatons who live by the 'clock'—wondering when the 14-day isolation is over, when curfew is over, and most importantly when this hardship is over." When the pandemic is over, continues Naguy, "those severely traumatized might suffer PTSD with flashbacks and nightmares as if reliving [the] experience at slightest reminder. Enduring personality changes might also ensue."

A survey conducted in Australia by the University of New South Wales in May 2020, and reported on The Conversation, found that when the first round of lockdowns was beginning to ease, one person in four said they were "very or extremely worried about contracting Covid-19." That by itself was not a sign of phobia, but according to the survey's leader, Jill Newby, when the fears and behaviors begin to gang up, when you find yourself wearing a mask and gloves when you're alone in your car, or you become overly diligent about cleaning and decontaminating your apartment, and you spend a lot of time checking your body for symptoms of infection, it may be time, Newby suggests, to "get help from professionals, not Dr. Google." Always good advice.

Above-the-Keyboard Dressing / *Choosing what to wear for online meetings while self-isolating, which means being concerned about your appearance solely from the waist up. Also called "desk dressing."*

For many of us, working from home during the pandemic meant dressing from the desk up, like television newscasters—impeccable above the waist, but perhaps wearing sweats and a pair of slippers below, where no one could see. I first heard the expression from a friend who owns a clothing store, where I'd gone to buy a shirt for an upcoming event. When I told her I didn't need a new pair of pants because the event was on Zoom, she said, "Ah, we call that 'above-the-keyboard dressing.'"

The phrase first appeared in March 2020 in a report published by wgsn (formerly the Worth Global Style Network), a uk-based fashion forecaster, that predicted "above-the-keyboard dressing" would be a growing part of our lives throughout the pandemic, when most business meetings, social events, and even family visits would be conducted online. House of Colour, a firm of image consultants also based in the uk, picked up on this as "a pivotal trend for 2020 as we grow increasingly reliant on screen based communications for sharing our life activities, events and for promoting professional and personal brands." Retail outlets offered proof: sales of tailored jackets, informal shirts and blouses, cosmetics, eyeglasses, and hair products rose sharply in 2020, while such "off-screen" accessories as pants, shoes, and handbags, deemed "less important," plummeted.

In July 2020, Bloomberg reported that "dress shoe sales may never recover to pre-Covid levels." In the us, sales of formal oxfords for men and high heels for women fell 71 percent in the second quarter of 2020, although overall footwear sales fell only 26 percent, bolstered as they were by increased sales of slippers and slides. The business suit firm Brooks Brothers filed for bankruptcy that month, followed by the Ascena

Retail Group, which owned the Ann Taylor brand of women's workwear.

Pants sales were down 13 percent, especially if they required belts (down 13 percent in the Asia-Pacific region, 22.1 percent in North America and Europe, and 24.1 percent in Latin America). Men's suspenders sales were also down 8 percent. "No one is buying pants," reported CNN, "but pajama sales are soaring." In the US, pajama sales rose 143 percent.

Sales of everyday purses and tote bags were down by 20 percent in July 2020, but high-end handbags did very well. In November, a Himalaya Kelly bag, touted by Luxuo as "the most desirable handbag in existence," sold at Christie's in Hong Kong for US$437,330. And in the US, the collection of socialite Susan Casden (for whom Hermès named "The Susan" handbag) sold for over $900,000. As the collector perceptively noted, no matter how bad things get, "people will still need to carry things."

People may always need to buy things too, especially after a prolonged period of consumer abstinence. That's the feeling of Amanda Mull, a staff writer at *The Atlantic*. Although she notes that "the pandemic has been tough on many types of businesses, but particularly on those peddling clothes," she adds that after previous pandemics, people rebounded with a heightened desire to dress well head to toe. "Some historians," she writes, "credit the plague for sparking demand for finely tailored clothing and luxury goods."

Think of the Renaissance finery after the retreat of the plague, when, as Carole Collier Frick writes in *Dressing Renaissance Florence*, wealthy Italians who survived the Black Death invested up to 40 percent of their fortunes in clothing. Wigs and heavy facial makeup became popular during the seventeenth century to cover the ravages of syphilis and smallpox. And after the 1918 influenza pandemic, "the country exploded into rebellion and exuberance," writes Mull. "Young women unlaced their corsets and opted for still-shorter hemlines." She predicts that when Covid restrictions are lifted, people will "be searching stores and their own closets for an answer to an unfamiliar question: What do you wear to reenter society?"

Apparently, they won't be searching the stores so much, at least not according to the website Fibre2Fashion. "The days of picking through the racks with your own two hands are over for now," the site says. During Covid, there was a significant drop in consumers' "intention to purchase." In the US and Europe, that drop was greater for in-store purchases (70 to 80 percent) than for online buying (30 to 40 percent), but it's clear that people are becoming fed up with what is called "fast fashion," or the "take-make-waste" approach to clothing ourselves.

Before Covid, 72 percent of the clothing sold was made from synthetic fibers that take up to two hundred years to decompose in landfill sites. Consumers indicate that they want, as well as buying less, to buy smarter: 60 percent say that environmental impact is now an important factor in deciding what to buy. The $1.5 trillion-a-year fashion industry is responding. The buzzword in the salons now is "circularity." To make it in the post-Covid market, reported *Forbes* magazine in January 2021, a new dress or a pair of shoes will need to have circularity, which means manufacturers will be "making sure resources and products stay in use for as long as possible before being regenerated into new products." What goes around comes around; in the 1970s and 1980s, we used to call that the three Rs: reduce, reuse, recycle. Consumers now say they intend to reduce, and companies are going to have to reuse and recycle.

Some companies are already responding. Nike now has a "Reuse-A-Shoe" program, which places drop-boxes in their stores in which customers can deposit their old shoes for recycling. Apple is offering to take back old computers that are still functional, and the European lingerie company Hunkemöller urges customers to return used lingerie so they can recycle the textiles. Many of these companies are finally realizing what those of us who remember the 1960s have been saying all along—that going green can actually increase profits. Subaru of Indiana Automotive decided a decade ago not to contribute anything to landfill sites: now they say they're saving $1.2 million a year.

It's unfortunate, of course, that it took 15 million deaths to wake up some corporations to the concept of environmental impact. But it's interesting that this new concern for the planet is consumer driven, and that (as we've always known) change doesn't come from the top down, but from the bottom up.

Quarantini / *Any alcoholic drink consumed during a lockdown.*

It didn't take long. As early as March 13, 2020, when the pandemic was just beginning to be felt in the US, the Novice Chef website posted a recipe for a quarantini cocktail. "You can't find toilet paper, everyone is stuck in the house from school and work and the whole family just got into a huge fight over your 100th game of Monopoly. What are you going to do?" the Novice Chef asks. "How about we make a Quarantini and chill!" The author then gives a recipe for a honey lemon martini, a concoction of vodka (or gin), lemon, honey, and water, with powdered vitamin C rimming the glass. It sounds more like a caipirinha to me, but as the Novice Chef says, you can throw anything you want into the shaker and call it a quarantini.

The photo accompanying the recipe shows a chilled cocktail glass beside a stack of toilet paper rolls, the inference being that in the early days of the pandemic, people stocked up on liquor as much as they hoarded toilet paper. That was the Covid Uncertainty Principle at work: we didn't know how long the lockdowns were going to last, we'd heard about problems with supply chains, and stores were running out of essential items, so we had better get in a good supply of everything. In March 2020, retail studies already showed that sales of alcohol had risen 17.5 percent in a single month, and in some places were 55 percent greater than in the same month in 2019. By December, *Forbes* reported that according to the marketing research company IWSR, which monitors the global alcohol trade, online sales of alcohol in 2020 had risen 80 percent. Total online sales of booze in the US rose from $3 billion in 2019 to $5.6 billion in a single year. Alcohol hadn't moved that well since the days of Prohibition.

And that was just online. Brick-and-mortar outlets were also recording record-breaking sales right into 2021. By then it was clear that the pandemic was not going away any time soon, and people were filling their cellars in anticipation of future shortages. Restaurants and bars might be closed at any time. Supply chains might snap. When governments shut down other retail outlets, they extended special "essential" status to liquor stores, as they did for grocery stores and pharmacies. Selling alcohol was an essential service. Going out to buy booze was essential travel. People needed to eat, drink, and take antidepressants. Several states allowed bars, restaurants, and even breweries and distilleries to deliver alcohol to people's homes, a service not included in statistics about e-commerce sales, which tracked only orders from local liquor stores made through phone apps. In New York City, many of those deliveries were made by a company called Drizly, which—shortly before it was bought by Uber for $1.1 billion—reported that its sales figures in 2020 were up 350 percent.

People weren't just hoarding alcohol; they were also drinking it. Among surveyed Australians, 70 percent said they were drinking more than they had been before the pandemic, 34 percent said they were drinking every day, and 20 percent said they were starting to drink earlier in the day. In a Harris poll conducted in the US from March 30 to April 7, 2020, 17 percent of respondents said they'd started drinking heavily since the beginning of the pandemic, and almost half of those reported that by "heavily," they meant five or more drinks a day. After noting that alcohol is the fourth leading preventable cause of death in America, a study published in December 2020 in the *International Journal of Environmental Research and Public Health* went on to say that 60 percent of respondents reported they were drinking more during the pandemic, citing higher stress levels, easy availability, and boredom as the three main reasons for their increased imbibing. (In the UK, a social agency called We Are With You gave another reason: support groups such as Alcoholics Anonymous were not available during the pandemic.) In one "large Midwest US healthcare system," the authors of the *IJERPH* study write, "the number of alcohol-related complaints, as a percentage of total behavioral health [emergency department]

visits, increased from 28.2 percent to 33.5 percent."
Hospitals whose emergency departments and ICUs
were already overburdened with Covid cases "may
not be able to continue responding to people who have
alcohol-related emergencies."

The rise in alcohol consumption may have contributed to the spread of Covid-19. "Alcohol consumption,"
warned the WHO in April 2020, "is associated with a
range of communicable and noncommunicable diseases
and mental health disorders, which can make a person
more vulnerable to Covid-19." Apart from the fact that
alcohol drinkers generally gather in large groups and
make bad decisions about face masks, social distancing,
and yelling, the WHO stated that "alcohol compro-
mises the body's immune system." A study conducted
in 2015 at Loyola University Chicago's departments of
medicine and public health found that after drinking
five shots of vodka, a person has a less active immune
system than when sober, making that person more
susceptible to respiratory infections. In reporting the
study's findings, the American Public Health Association added that, at the time, one in six American adults
binge-drank an average of four times a month, and that
"more than half of the alcohol consumed in the US [is]
drunk in the form of binge drinking." Those figures
rose sharply during the first year of the pandemic.

Liquor sales have trailed off since that early wave of
bottled oblivion. During the week of March 6–13, 2021,
liquor sales in the US actually went down 1.9 percent.

They were still well over 2019 levels, but no longer soaring. I suspect the drop in off-sale purchases and home deliveries was not the result of sober reflection or health concerns on the part of the general public; I suspect it was because by March, the bars had reopened.

Covidivorce / *A parting of ways arising from a couple's prolonged close confinement during the pandemic.*

"Couples whose marriages are fraying under the pressures of self-isolation could be heading for a 'covidivorce,'" cautioned the *New York Times* in March 2020. The authors cited reports from China, where lengthy lockdowns were imposed early and "the number of divorce applications surged... in at least two Chinese provinces, Sichuan and Shanxi... as altercations intensified between quarantined couples." The *Times* subsequently added "covidivorce" to its lexicon, and the Collins Dictionary considered adding the word as well, as divorces and inquiries about divorces to us lawyers increased by more than 35 percent during the pandemic's first year. In the UK, the BBC reported that from July to October 2020 divorce inquiries shot 122 percent above the same period in 2019.

This upsurge (not just an uptick) has apparently not happened in Canada, where the divorce rate has remained steady at around 70,000 per year, with 40 percent of marriages ending in divorce before the couple's thirtieth anniversary. A survey conducted by the Vanier Institute of the Family found that nearly 80 percent of responders aged eighteen or older said they and their spouses were supporting one another well during the pandemic, and Statistics Canada reports that although the number of divorces has been increasing in Canada since 2000, it increased in 2020 at the same rate as it had in the past two decades.

Inquiries surged in the US in 2020, but the actual divorce rate hasn't risen since 1990. That may be because fewer people are getting married. Among those who do marry, reports the *New York Times* (March 24, 2021), "the uncertainty of the pandemic and financial concerns are two reasons couples are staying together." In other words, couples may be staying together not because they think their relationship is working but because their financial situation has changed and they can't afford to get divorced. For them, the pandemic has made the future look grimmer than the prospect of staying with an unsuitable partner. (It's rather like living in a Henry James novel.)

Femicide / *The killing of a woman by her male partner or former partner, an extreme form of intimate partner violence (IPV) that has increased significantly as lockdowns and isolation policies have been implemented during the pandemic.*

In France, on the first day of 2022, three women were murdered by their male partners or former partners. In that country in 2021, 113 women had been killed by their partners, and in Europe 600 others were similarly murdered, an increase from 444 in 2020. "The number of femicides from year to year is not falling," said Marylie Breuil, a spokesperson for NousToutes, a women's group in France lobbying for stricter laws relating to domestic violence. Breuil added that two-thirds of the dead women had reported being abused by their partners to the police, and no action had been taken.

Incidents of IPV increased everywhere during the pandemic. In Canada, BC human rights commissioner Kasari Govender warned in April 2020 that "in these times of great stress in society, violence will go up, especially behind closed doors... In BC, we see that evidenced through the increased demand for services, for anti-violence services. One service provider [Vancouver's Battered Women's Support Services] reported a 300 percent increase in calls over this time."

Canadian lawyer Pamela Cross, who specializes in cases of violence against women, writes in the *Lawyer's Daily* (March 18, 2020) that self-isolation has had unique impacts on vulnerable populations, especially on women in abusive relationships who are isolated with their partners and unable to distance themselves from interpersonal violence. "With increased social isolation, a woman is more vulnerable to her partner's emotional and physical abuse," writes Cross, noting that during periods of lockdown, with the closing of workplaces, schools, libraries, community centers, arenas, and services such as women's shelters, "the current public health crisis is a gift to abusers."

A national survey conducted from May 18 to July 20, 2020, by the Ending Violence Association of Canada found that victims of domestic violence were generally less able to access programs or seek help during the pandemic. For example, the Sudbury Women's Centre, which in pre-Covid days helped 150 to 200 women at any given time, saw a significant drop in clients after coronavirus restrictions were imposed. From May to July, only thirty-five women came to the center. The survey found that domestic abusers learned to change their tactics; they took advantage of the pandemic to increase control over their victims, used information about Covid-19 to isolate their partners, and limited access to the phones and computers that would have enabled women to contact social agencies or even friends.

Across Canada and the US, police departments reported an increase of 12 percent in calls related to domestic violence between March and June 2020. The Assaulted Women's Helpline, a free, anonymous telephone line open to Ontario women, reported that from April to December 2020 the agency received 71,633 calls, an increase of nearly 100 percent over 2019.

On November 25, 2021—International Day for the Elimination of Violence Against Women—the Canadian Femicide Observatory for Justice and

Accountability reported that ninety-two women and girls had been killed in Canada between January and June of that year, an increase from seventy-eight during the same six months of 2020 and sixty in the same period in 2019.

"Canada is not the only country experiencing these continual increases in numbers," University of Guelph researcher Myrna Dawson told CTV News. "It's a global trend."

Indeed it is. In Germany in 2021, a woman was killed by her male partner every two and a half days. In January 2021, Puerto Rican governor Pedro Pierluisi declared a state of emergency because of an increase in femicides: sixty women in 2020, a 60 percent jump over 2019. And Mexico recorded the most alarming statistics of all. In January 2022, Amnesty International released the report *Justice on Trial*, stating that at least ten women had been killed in Mexico every day in 2020. Not all of them had been victims of their male partners, but of the 3,723 cases of murdered women that year, 940 were investigated as femicides. Although the crime rate in Mexico overall dropped by 10 percent that year, femicides increased by 7.1 percent and rapes by 30 percent. Wendy Figueroa, director of the National Network of Shelters in Mexico, points to the isolation resulting from the pandemic as a major factor in the increase. "Governments forgot the gender perspective," she told the website Atalayar on June 29, 2021, "and left women locked up with their aggressors."

The United Nations defined "femicide" in 2012 as "the killing of women and girls because of their gender." But only Argentina and Chile differentiate femicides from other types of homicide. Since those separate statistics have been kept, the incidence of femicide has declined in both countries.

Shecession / *A pandemic-related recession in which those most affected are women.*

Pandemic closures put many people out of work and obliged others to work from home. In both cases, the *New York Times* reported in June 2020, "the economic fallout from the pandemic is threatening to derail the careers of an entire generation of working women." More than half (55 percent) of the 20.5 million jobs lost in the US that month had been held by women, a disappointing reversal from December 2019, when for the first time since the Great Depression women had held more payroll jobs—that is, excluding household and farm jobs—than men. By the end of June 2020, 16.5 percent of working women were unemployed, compared with 15 percent of working men. In September 2020, 863,000 women dropped out of the labor force, compared to 168,000 men. And Shelley Zalis reports in *Forbes* that "of the 150,000 jobs lost in December 2020, all belonged to women." All of which prompted C. Nicole Mason, president and CEO of the Institute for

Women's Policy Research, to remark, "We should go ahead and call this a 'shecession.'"

Lurking within the larger picture were data showing that most of the jobs lost by women were in hospitality and health care. These jobs were held primarily by immigrants and women of color, and few if any of them could be done at home. The Representation Project, an initiative started in 2011 to counter gender stereotyping, notes that "women of color have had the sharpest declines to their employment-to-population ratios... in a one month span. From February to April 2020, Black, Asian, and Latina women suffered larger losses to their employment ratio than white women." This means that a higher percentage of women of color lost their jobs than white women.

In March 2021, Canadian finance minister Chrystia Freeland announced the formation of the Task Force on Women in the Economy—which she would cochair with associate finance minister Mona Fortier—to address ways in which the federal budget for 2021 could help offset the imbalance between jobs lost by women and those lost by men. One suggestion was to establish a nationwide childcare system. To that end, the 2021 federal budget included $27.2 billion toward "bringing fees for regulated child care down to $10 per day on average within the next five years."

The problems specific to immigrant women and women of color were also on the table. Panel member Maya Roy, chief executive officer of YWCA Canada, said that reaching out to unemployed immigrant women whose training was not recognized in Canada was a priority: "There are highly trained women out there who are delivering pizzas and driving Ubers."

Justin Trudeau, who campaigned on the issue of feminism and gender equality, said that "this crisis has created a shecession and has threatened to roll back the hard-fought social and economic progress of all women... To build a fairer and more equal Canada, we must ensure a feminist, intersectional recovery from the crisis."

The reasons for the disproportionate effects of the pandemic on racialized women, however, are the same as those for their marginalized status in the population at large: sexism, racism, and discriminatory social policies. The shecession is another way in which the pandemic has underlined systemic flaws in the social system, inequalities that have been there all along. "The fact is," writes Jaime Watt in the May 24, 2020, issue of the *Toronto Star*, "these issues did not arrive with Covid-19 nor will they disappear with a vaccine."

Corona Bonds / *Proposed bonds to be issued by the European Investment Bank to raise funds to pay off debts incurred by European Union member states during the pandemic; essentially a means of spreading one country's debt across the entire European Union.*

Issuing such mutualized bonds would be a reversal of the EU's policy, according to which the Union cannot be held liable for debts incurred by individual members.

The debate about corona bonds was between poorer southern countries—including Spain, Italy, Greece, Portugal, and Slovenia—where the coronavirus was more devastating and the economic impact more disastrous—and the wealthier northern states, such as Germany, the Netherlands, Austria, and Finland, where the virus had been less heavily felt and the national economies were not yet almost-beyond recovery.

On April 23, 2020, when Italian prime minister Giuseppe Conte requested an immediate rescue package of 1.5 trillion euros, the nineteen EU ministers of finance proposed an alternative solution: that the European Stability Mechanism (ESM)—an international financial institution based in Luxembourg set up to make emergency loans available to EU member states—provide half a trillion euros to EU nations in the form of loans or repayable grants and that the European Investment Bank (EIB) make more loan guarantees available to struggling companies in cash-strapped countries.

But there would be no "corona bonds." In fact, in reports of the meeting, the phrase "corona bonds" did not even come up. As specified in the EU constitution, individual nations are responsible for their own economies, and their debts will not be shared by all member countries. "Pooling European debt would have been a near-impossible feat as it faced resistance from the region's richer countries," as Bloomberg observed.

By June 2021, however, even the wealthier nations were struggling to meet the financial demands of the pandemic, largely because they had incurred massive debt loads. Germany's 2021 budget projected borrowing 240 billion euros, a record high that pushed its overall national debt to 2.2 trillion euros. In response to the general malaise, the EU issued ten-year "debut bonds" with more or less the same aim corona bonds would have had: to address union members' debt issues. The bonds raised 20 billion euros in the first two weeks and were expected to raise another 80 billion by the end of the year. These funds, along with the 750 billion euro Covid recovery fund, would still be made available to member countries, only in the form of loans. Still no corona bonds.

Eurostat, the EU's statistical agency, reported that for EU member nations the average debt ratio—the amount of debt in relation to the country's gross domestic product—was 100 percent, which meant most countries were borrowing about the same amount as the value of the goods they produced. But there was still the north-south divide: despite its record debt, Germany's debt ratio was 80 percent, whereas Greece's was 200 percent and Italy's was 180 percent. The southern nations, however, could still expect little relief from the EU. Markus Ferber, a financial expert with Germany's Christian Social Union party, told the German news website DW in October 2021 that "those who think they can restructure their national budget by shifting the mountains of debt to Europe will fail... These will eventually have to be paid off by the member states."

This decision seemed to contradict the EU's much-vaunted notion that "we're all in this together." The division between have and have-not economies was as clear as it had been in the days before the Union.

Corona Corridor / *An arrangement that allowed for-eign visitors from a country with low Covid cases to travel through another country without submitting to that country's quarantine or self-isolation protocols, and return to their native country without having to be quarantined.*

In late April 2020, the Czech Republic announced plans to issue "health certificates" to travelers coming into the Czech Republic from Austria and Slovenia en route to Croatia and the Adriatic coast. The European tourism industry expected to lose 12 billion euros that year, and Croatia was one of hardest hit even though, at the time, it had recorded only thirty-three Covid deaths. Cases in the UK were in decline, and so Croa-tia suggested issuing health certificates to travelers entering from there. But, as Krunoslav Capak, head of the Croatian Institute for Public Health, warned, "Health certificates do not mean much because a person may be ill twenty-four hours later."

In May, as Greece's financial problems mounted, the Greek government also contemplated opening borders to travelers from countries that had Covid under control. With Greece acting as a corona corridor for Cyprus and Israel, vacationers would have access to Greek islands in the Aegean and Mediterranean by early July. "It is an ambitious scheme that could square the circle," said Harry Theoharis, Greece's minister for tourism, perhaps forgetting that squaring the circle had been considered impossible by Greek mathematicians since the days of Pythagoras. Did he perhaps mean that wealthy tourists visiting Athens would be able to circle the square?

In the fall, as Covid numbers began climbing again, the UK ended its flirtation with corona corridors by adding Croatia to its list of countries from which British travelers would have to quarantine for fourteen days upon their return to Britain. On August 18, when there were an estimated 20,000 British citizens in Croatia, the country recorded 219 Covid cases. The UK had already put Spain on its quarantine list and was closely watching Greece, Denmark, the Faroe Islands, Austria, Switzerland, and Gibraltar.

No island is an island during a pandemic, however, and despite these belated stabs at isolation, Britain's

Covid cases continued to rise, averaging about 1,500 new cases a day, and soaring to nearly 60,000 a day in January 2021. Indulging in corona corridors had not been a good idea.

Coronnial; Coronababy / *A child conceived and/or born during the pandemic.*

In March 2020, a *New York Times* article noted that "the crisis has spawned a new lexicon. Where once there were 'blackout babies,' we can now expect a wave of 'coronababies.' " *Esquire* described a coronnial as one "practically born wearing [a] face shield." In April, Global News wondered "if extra time in lockdown will lead to a new generation of 'coronnials.' "

If it does, it won't be because time spent in lockdown meant more women became pregnant. In the US, where the birth rate has been falling for years, the decline during the pandemic became more pronounced. There were about 40,000 fewer births at the end of 2020 than had been expected. During the last three months of the year, the birth rate was 53.9 births per thousand women, down from 57.6 per thousand in the last quarter of 2019. The biggest decline was in women between the ages of fifteen and twenty-four, suggesting that perhaps fewer people were able to form couples during the pandemic. In parts of Europe, the decline was even steeper. A study of fertility plans in Europe showed that 50 percent of couples in Germany and France who had planned to have a child in 2020 had decided to postpone; in Italy, 37 percent decided not to have children at all, ever. And Spain experienced a 20 percent drop in its birth rate, the largest decline since the country began keeping records.

A number of reasons for the baby bust have been proposed. People isolated in their homes, not socializing, was cited as a big factor. Loss of income was another. Historically, noted the BBC in December 2020, "economic confidence has led to a rise in births and uncertainty to a decline." And studies do show that the decline in births is more pronounced in the areas of Europe and North America whose economies were most negatively affected by the pandemic.

There is also evidence that pregnant women are slightly more susceptible to Covid-19 than women who are not, and knowing this may have acted as a deterrent to becoming pregnant. Resistance to Covid-19 depends on a strong immune response, and the immune systems of pregnant women adapt slightly downward to allow for the growth of the fetus, which, since it shares only half its DNA with the mother, would be at risk of rejection if the immune system were working at full capacity.

Pregnant women who have Covid-19 may also have a higher likelihood of placental abnormalities. A study at Northwestern University reported a higher incidence of maternal vascular malperfusion (MVM)—a condition associated with stillbirth, premature birth, and reduced fetal growth—among births to women who have Covid-19. And physicians in China reported higher incidence of chorangiosis, perivillous fibrin, and multiple villous infarcts—all of which come from interruptions in the blood supply to the placenta— among pregnant women infected with the disease.

Some long-term physical and psychological effects of being born during the pandemic may not become apparent for years. A 2014 study conducted at McGill University and the Douglas Mental Health University Institute examined 180 children who'd been born in Montreal during the ice storm of 1998, when pregnant women were isolated in their homes for weeks. They found that thirty-six of them (20 percent) showed greater risk of asthma, diabetes, and obesity, and also displayed minor developmental delays in IQ, motor skills, and bilateral coordination, or the ability to coordinate both sides of their body during an activity.

Changes in the women's T cells (the cells responsible for activating the immune system and metabolizing sugar) resulted from "objective stress exposure" in the mothers—sudden and prolonged changes in routine, such as having no electricity for forty-five days and not knowing when the ordeal would end—rather than from the kind of emotional stress created by longer-term factors, such as poverty or the threat of domestic violence. A pregnant woman who does not know when or if a situation is going to improve appears to pass more stress to the fetus than she herself experiences, which is why Suzanne King, a psychopathologist at McGill and Douglas who was involved in the 2014 study, advised women who became pregnant during lockdowns in the early days of Covid-19 to "try to stay as positive as possible."

Objective stress exposure seems assured during a pandemic, when there is no way to know how long restrictions will last, whether there will be another wave, another variant, or another shutdown, and no amount of assurance from government or health officials seems to make a difference. In the Before Times, psychologists argued that all stress is subjective, but during the pandemic much of what psychologists said went out the window.

Covid Zero / *The state of a population with no cases of Covid-19.*

"Some people have gotten this idea that we're going to get to 'Covid Zero,' " Dr. Amesh Adalja, of Johns Hopkins University, told the *New York Times* on February 24, 2021. "That's not realistic. It's a fantasy."

In January 2021, the editors of the journal *Nature* asked one hundred epidemiologists, virologists, and infectious disease researchers whether in their view Covid-19 could ever be eradicated. "Almost 90 percent of respondents," reports Nicky Phillips in a *Nature* news feature February 16, "think that the coronavirus will... continue to circulate in pockets of the global population for years to come." They expect that Covid-19 will become endemic, turning up in one form or another in perpetuity, like influenza. Extirpation may be possible, but not extinction. As one respondent put it, trying to eradicate coronavirus is "like trying to plan the construction of a stepping-stone pathway to the moon."

There are, of course, those who disagree. Some governments adopted a strategy they called Go for Zero, or #CovidZero, involving the complete shutdown of borders, businesses, schools, and other public places, combined with rigid restrictions against travel and social gathering, until health authorities in those areas reported zero new cases for a significant length of time. In effect, Covid Zero was an active way of trying to achieve herd immunity. And for a while, in some countries, it looked as though it might work.

In July 2020, Australia, under the government of Scott Morrison, and following a recommendation by the Grattan Institute, a public policy think tank, announced it was going to "go for zero" rather than try to flatten the curve. As well as closing businesses and schools, the government imposed a nighttime curfew, forbade citizens to travel more than five kilometers (three miles) from their homes, and imposed fines for breaking the rules. In some districts, police conducted spot checks and arrested anti-restriction protesters.

The state of Victoria also designated "health hotels," or "hot hotels," for the use of arriving travelers who tested positive for the virus.

By September 2020, new cases had decreased enough that some restrictions were lifted. During the last week in December, the country reported only ten new cases a day (down from seven hundred in August), and between October and December there was only one Covid-related death.

Australia was following the example of New Zealand, whose prime minister, Jacinda Ardern, had imposed strict restrictions in February 2020, including border closures and a ban on travel; in early June, the country reported zero active cases of Covid-19. An analysis published by *The Lancet* later showed that of the 1,503 cases in New Zealand between February 2 and May 13, 2020, 575 had been imported by travelers and 459 were tracked to people who had had contact with those travelers, showing that closing the borders, followed by efficient contact tracing, was a highly effective way to reduce cases.

Atlantic Canada adopted a "Go for Zero" policy in December 2020. Dr. Andrew Morris, writing in the *Canadian Medical Association Journal*, called on the federal government to refocus Canada's pandemic response to more closely resemble the policy in the Atlantic region, urging policy makers to try to eliminate the virus rather than simply manage it with on-again, off-again measures. Elimination, according to Morris, was the best way to avoid wave after wave of lockdowns, restrictions, and renewed surges of infection. And he initiated a campaign called #CovidZero to rally Canadians to the Go for Zero cause.

Andrew Nikiforuk, author of *Pandemonium*, agreed with Morris, writing in the BC publication *The Tyee* that trying to manage the virus would not work because organizing a managerial response always took longer than the virus needed to mutate, ensuring a constant stream of new variants. He advocated a complete shutdown of everything, with travel restrictions between countries, provinces, and even regions, as well as "brief and decisive localized lockdowns followed by an aggressive program of find/test/trace/isolate/support," as had proven effective in New Zealand and Atlantic Canada. The biggest ally of the pandemic, he said, was complacency. "If you want to fail and live through a third wave," he wrote, "just wait for the vaccine. If not, then flood your politicians with one message: Go to zero."

Total lockdowns seemed to work for a time, but in the end, keeping the pandemic outside the gates proved impossible. There were too many Trojan horses, and too many variants. It was the Delta variant that ended New Zealand's isolation policy. On October 4, 2021, after a year and a half of insisting on Covid Zero, Jacinda Ardern called a halt to closures and restrictions. They hadn't kept Covid out and had finally exhausted the population's endurance. After 200,000 people demonstrated against continued lockdown in Auckland, Ardern announced that "for this outbreak, it's clear that long periods of heavy restrictions have not got us to zero cases."

The problem in New Zealand was a lack of vaccinations, particularly for the Māori community. "The PM says we must now live with the virus," tweeted Morgan Godfery, a Māori writer and community leader. "But the 'we' means these same lines of inequality. The virus will now burrow in gangs, the transitional housing community, and unvaccinated brown people."

Epidemiologists and Māori leaders encouraged Ardern to hang on to lockdowns, hoping she would continue with restrictions until a larger percentage of the overall population had been vaccinated. But Ardern recognized that most New Zealanders had had enough. On October 5, 2021, when New Zealand was recording about forty new cases a day, Ardern went beyond her earlier "social bubble" recommendations and allowed households to meet with other households outdoors, in parks, and on beaches—and sent younger children back to school. By the end of October, new cases had shot up to an average of 130 per day, and the curve was not flattening.

One of the reasons Ardern had responded so quickly to the Covid pandemic may have been the memory of the 1918 influenza pandemic. New Zealand had been slow to respond, allowing ships from infected countries to dock in the harbor at Auckland. Within three months, more than 11,500 New Zealanders had died and the disease had spread into half a dozen southeast Asian countries trading with New Zealand. It seems that even those who know their history are condemned to repeat it.

Emergency Brake / *The sudden application of strict social and economic measures to halt the spread of Covid.*

"Emergency brake" is a dubious metaphor for total lockdown, since, in cars, the emergency brake is applied only when the vehicle is already stopped. However, the term was employed by Ontario premier Doug Ford on April 3, 2021, to characterize his government's new health measures, which put the province into a six-week lockdown in response to the third Covid wave. "The Ontario government," read the media release, "is imposing a provincewide emergency brake as a result of an alarming surge in case numbers and Covid-19 hospitalizations across the province." Shutdown measures, similar to restrictions applied in January 2021 during the second Covid wave, prohibited outdoor public events and social gatherings and limited the capacity of indoor private events to a five-person maximum. Restaurants could offer only curbside pickup, drive-through, and delivery—no more of those individually sealed sidewalk incubators. Gyms, ball-parks, and fitness centers were closed. Originally, schools were allowed to remain open, but within weeks pupils were sent home with online learning packages, and in-person teaching did not resume for the remainder of the school year.

None of these measures were new and when put in place before had raised little alarm. What caused a backlash this time was the provision that gave police the power to stop motorists and pedestrians to ensure that they were engaged in "essential" activities, such as shopping for food or medicine (or alcohol), attending medical appointments, or "exercising outdoors with members of their household." Anyone found away from their homes for a nonessential reason could be fined, and refusal to provide information when asked by police was deemed a crime punishable by imprisonment.

Civil rights groups in the province quickly pointed out the danger of such legislation. "Ontario is one step closer to becoming a police state," warned the executive director of the Canadian Constitution Foundation. Warren Thomas, president of the Ontario Public Service Employees Union (OPSEU), said that "to give the police the right to stop and question citizens is akin to martial law."

The situation was resolved, after a fashion, when Chief Nishan Duraiappah of Peel Regional Police told

Global News on April 17 that "our officers will not be conducting random vehicle or individual stops." Within a week, police departments around the province made similar announcements, and on April 20, the stop-and-question part of the lockdown order was rescinded.

Giving police extraordinary powers and hoping they don't use them does not make for a civil society, and this erosion of the democratic process, although quickly averted, invited comparison with countries in which civil liberties were threatened. During the pandemic, governments around the world enacted legislation to restrict freedom of movement, freedom of association, and freedom of expression by invoking the name of Covid—worldwide, 138 countries, including many with democratic governments, enacted more than three hundred new laws using the pandemic as a pretext for clamping down on citizens' rights.

Italian police were authorized to disperse people on the streets—not just protesters, but anyone. French citizens needed signed *passes sanitaires* to leave their homes. In Israel, the cell phones of citizens who tested positive for Covid were tracked to make sure their owners were obeying quarantine orders. China, already in the process of using facial recognition technology and WeChat to monitor citizens, added thermal cameras to track infected people. Would these measures be dismantled when the pandemic passed? Or would they be kept in place and used to locate and arrest dissidents?

If freedom of movement and association can be policed, what about freedom of speech and freedom of expression? In January 2021, the Organisation for Economic Co-operation and Development noted that "in the first nine months of the pandemic, over forty-four countries enacted new laws or decrees that chill speech, including many that impose criminal penalties for the dissemination of 'fake news' about the pandemic." Often "fake news" means "views that don't coincide with those of the authorities." Covid-19 "has also given governments such as Egypt's an excuse to crack down on their critics," noted *The Economist* in February, "using the pretext of restricting the spread of fake news."

In June 2020, Egyptian journalist Mohamed Monir, who had appeared on Al Jazeera criticizing the Egyptian government's response to the pandemic, was arrested for spreading "false news," misusing social media, and belonging to "a terrorist group." He was one of six journalists held in Egypt's infamous Tora Prison; while incarcerated, he contracted Covid-19 and died two weeks after his arrest.

CIVICUS Monitor, a civil rights watchdog organization that produces regularly updated data on freedom of peaceful assembly and the Covid-19 pandemic, noted in December 2020 that 87 percent of the world's population lived in countries where civil liberties are "closed, repressed, or obstructed." Its lead researcher, Marianna Belalba Barreto, decried "the hypocrisy of governments using Covid-19 as a pretense to crack down on protests." Just as corporations use a recession as an excuse to make staff and payroll cuts they had intended to make anyway, so governments take advantage of crises in order to seize control of a citizenry.

Hero Pay / *Bonus pay offered to employees for continuing to work during the pandemic. Also called hazard pay, thank-you pay, appreciation pay, or service pay.*

On March 4, 2021, the US government passed legislation to provide funding for frontline workers who become ill as a result of working closely with Covid patients during the pandemic. Called the Pandemic Heroes Compensation Act, it set aside $10 billion spread over ten years to be paid to "essential workers," either as bonuses or as compensation for their Covid-related medical expenses.

Somehow, the combination of the word "heroes" in the title of the act and the mention of "essential workers" in the literature accompanying it led many people to believe that private companies that provided "essential" services during the pandemic, and paid their employees a bonus to keep coming to work despite the danger of being exposed to Covid, made their employees "heroes" and the extra compensation was to be called "hero pay." Some companies designated as essential—grocery stores and pharmacies—did pay their checkout clerks slightly higher wages. Other companies that were less obviously essential, such as Starbucks, Walmart, Target, and Amazon, announced in mid-March 2020 that they'd pay employees an extra two or three dollars an hour for continuing to work during lockdowns. The bonuses were meant to be temporary, terminating at the end of May, but some companies extended them to the end of June, or until restrictions were lifted and it was safe for all employees to return to work.

The suggestion that Starbucks baristas were "heroes" for defying self-isolation guidelines stuck in the craw of some people. In "A Good Idea Goes Viral," an essay promoting universal basic income for vulnerable communities, Jamie Swift and Elaine Power note that the true heroes of the pandemic were the paramedics and personal service workers (PSWS) in long-term care facilities who, before Covid-19, were "invisible, taken for granted and poorly paid," and who continued to work even while the people for whom they provided care were dying around them. Swift and Power cite Miranda Ferrier of the Canadian Support Workers Association, who described the devastation felt by low-wage workers in long-term care institutions. "PSWS are crying before they go in for their shifts in long-term care. They cry in their cars."

"The idea of labelling it 'hero pay,'" writes Sylvain Charlebois in *Canadian Grocer* in June 2020, "was never going to end well." The Empire Company's grocery chain called it a "lockdown bonus," which was more accurate. The idea was not to reward heroes but to lure reluctant employees to work during stay-at-home restrictions, when new Covid cases were rising and working in close contact with the public was hazardous. Many employees refused to do it. "We didn't call it hero pay," a clerk at my local supermarket told me. "We called it danger pay. People were asked to risk their lives for two dollars an hour."

In the US, retail clerks made similar comments. An employee at a small grocery store in Wisconsin told NPR in May 2020 that an extra two dollars an hour hardly made a difference in her financial budget. "I don't think two dollars an hour is—hero pay?" she said. Especially when someone on unemployment was receiving six hundred dollars a week. "That's almost the whole paycheck for me," she said. "Even with hazard pay, I still don't make that much money." Columbia University economist Suresh Naidu said that hazard pay should be ten times what was being offered to essential workers.

In *Canadian Grocer*, Charlebois explained that grocery chains ended the hero pay program in May because Covid fears were "slowly fading away," and without the fear of infection, "the need to incentivize employees to show up for work" also disappeared. He noted that even large grocery chains operated on marginal profits, and raising employees' wages by two dollars an hour (representing a 10–15 percent increase in salaries) "made the average store almost unprofitable."

In the US, "hero pay" as provided by the Pandemic Heroes Compensation Act was more clearly understood as bonuses given to health-care workers and public employees who dealt with the fallout from Covid every day. In June 2021, when the Minnesota legislature allocated $250 million in hero pay to state frontline workers, employee organizations called it "a good first step" but pointed out that longer-term recognition would have been more welcome. "Bonuses are for bankers," Mary C. Turner, president of the Minnesota Nurses Association told the *Pioneer Press*. "This is backpay. This is making up for what we lost in pay and benefits while sitting in quarantine or waiting for tests."

In February 2021, the city council of Los Angeles voted in favor of requiring all grocery stores in L.A. with at least three hundred employees nationwide to raise their employees' salaries by five dollars an hour. Although L.A. mayor Eric Garcetti said that that shouldn't raise food prices "because grocery stores are one area that have record profits," by September, food prices in L.A. had risen an average of 4.6 percent.

Lab-Leak Theory / *The theory that the coronavirus responsible for Covid-19 originated in a laboratory in the Wuhan Institute of Virology (WIV) and somehow escaped from there into the general population; an alternative to the theory that the virus spilled over from bats to humans in the Huanan Seafood Market in Wuhan.*

On February 6, 2020, Botao Xiao, a Chinese virologist who had worked in the WIV before moving to the South China University of Technology, published a paper in a non-peer-reviewed journal in which he claimed that "the killer coronavirus probably originated from a laboratory in Wuhan." He cited only anecdotal evidence: there had been incidents of mishandled pathogens in other Chinese labs, and one of the researchers in Wuhan collected bats and was sometimes bitten by them. In response, two dozen international virologists signed a letter to *The Lancet* saying that "conspiracy theories do nothing but create fear, rumours, and prejudice that jeopardise our global collaboration in the fight against this virus." Botao withdrew his paper and apologized.

Supporting Botao's lab-leak theory, however, was a series of four papers coauthored in 2020 by Chinese virologist Li-Meng Yan claiming that in 2015 Chinese scientists, attempting to develop a bioweapon to conquer the world, genetically engineered the coronavirus that caused Covid-19. Li-Meng further claimed that "this virus came from the People's Liberation Army lab... and it was intentionally released."

The lab-leak theory, which was quickly picked up by Tom Cotton (the Republican senator from Arkansas), morphed in various tabloids—as well as in Donald Trump's press briefings—into a conviction that the virus was developed as part of China's bioweapons program and deliberately released to kill Americans.

Li-Meng Yan's credibility was challenged and the lab-leak theory discredited by the world scientific community. It had enough traction, however, that in February 2021, the WHO sent a ten-person team of investigators to Wuhan to determine where the coronavirus had originated and how it had spread to humans. Although the team met with resistance from Chinese authorities, its report confirmed that it was "extremely unlikely" that the virus had originated in the WIV lab. The WHO's own director-general, Tedros Adhanom Ghebreyesus, questioned those findings, saying that a deeper investigation was needed and that the lab-leak theory had not been adequately resolved.

In response to the WHO report, eighteen scientists wrote to the journal *Science* calling for further investigation, saying that both theories were "viable." Five other scientists, led by Dr. Kristian Andersen of Scripps Research, said that "our analyses clearly show that SARS-CoV-2 is not a laboratory construct or a purposefully manipulated virus." This seemed to close the door on the lab-leak theory; the majority scientific opinion was that the coronavirus had been transmitted naturally from bats to some intermediary animal at the Huanan Seafood Market, and from that mystery animal into humans.

Then, in May 2021, an article appeared in the *Bulletin of the Atomic Scientists* by Nicholas Wade, who had worked as an editor at both *Nature* and *Science*, and was a former science writer for the *New York Times*. Wade set out to "sort through the available scientific facts" behind the controversy. He began by casting doubt on the reliability of the two letters that had appeared in *The Lancet* and the journal *Nature Medicine* which had discredited the lab-leak theory. The *Lancet* letter, he wrote, had been organized and drafted by Peter Daszak, president of EcoHealth Alliance in New York—an institution that had connections with the Wuhan Institute of Virology. Daszak had been one of the scientists on the WHO team that had deemed it "extremely unlikely" that the virus had originated in the WIV lab. Wade thought that Daszak's involvement in the WHO report was therefore a conflict of interest.

The WIV researcher who collected bats in Botao's account was Shi Zhengli, a virologist known to her colleagues as "Bat Woman." She didn't collect bats; she collected bat serum that contained coronaviruses. In 2015, she teamed with University of North Carolina professor Ralph S. Baric and, according to Wade, "focused on enhancing the ability of bat viruses to attack humans." These "gain-of-function" experiments are common, designed to determine what virus characteristics are needed for a bat coronavirus to infect humans. Most of the thirty-two level 4 virology labs around the world—including Canada's National Microbiology Laboratory (NML) in Winnipeg—engage in similar work on a variety of infectious diseases. According to Wade, what Shi Zhengli was doing in her lab was taking an older strain of a bat coronavirus, such as the one responsible for SARS, and genetically engineering it to be more transmissible to humans. She then exposed "humanized mice" to it—lab mice that had, in their turn, been genetically modified to have human ACE2 receptors in their lungs. It was Shi Zhengli's modified SARS coronavirus, says Wade, that either escaped or was released from the WIV lab and caused the ensuing pandemic. That was why no bat had been found in the wild with SARS-COV-2, and no intermediate animal had been found in the Wuhan wet market: the intermediate animal was a humanized mouse in the WIV lab.

After the appearance of Wade's article, NIH director Dr. Francis Collins told the *New York Times* that "it is most likely that this is a virus that arose naturally, but we cannot exclude the possibility of some kind of a lab accident." Dr. Anthony Fauci, head of the NIAID, agreed: "I think we should continue to investigate what went on in China." A few days later, President Biden instructed the US intelligence community to assess whether the pandemic had "emerged from human contact with an infected animal or from a laboratory accident," and to report to him in ninety days.

Dr. Shi denies that she was engaged in gain-of-function research and that the pandemic originated in her lab. However, according to the *Guardian Weekly* (June 18, 2021), "of all the known bat coronaviruses, the most similar to SARS-CoV-2, sharing 96 percent of its genome, is RaTG13, a virus that researchers at the WIV were studying prior to the pandemic." Since then, however, other bat coronaviruses close to the SARS-CoV-2 virus have been found, including a cluster in the Chinese province of Yunnan, where Dr. Shi habitually collected her specimens.

Elaine Dewar's highly persuasive account of the controversy, *On the Origin of the Deadliest Pandemic in 100 Years*, presents compelling evidence in support of a lab leak, but even she admits there is no smoking gun. The most compelling evidence is still circumstantial: the secretiveness of the Chinese government, the fact that all level 4 labs in the world are engaged in gain-of-function research, the assumption that accidental leaks occur. Even Biden's security team, like the WHO delegation before it, came up empty-handed after its ninety-day search through whatever documentation they could find on the activities of the WIV.

In an article in the November 18, 2021, issue of *Science*, Michael Worobey of the University of Arizona presents an analysis of the question of Covid-19's origins. Worobey concludes that the first case of Covid-19 was that of a woman who worked as a seafood vendor in the Huanan Seafood Market. She developed symptoms on December 10, 2019, and had no connection at all with the Wuhan Institute of Virology. Most virologists now agree that the pandemic started in the wet market, not in a lab at the WIV.

Long-Hauler / *A patient whose Covid-19 symptoms persist for more than three weeks. "Long-hauler" and "long Covid" are the terms preferred by patients who have the disease; to medical professionals, it's known as "post-acute sequelae" (PASC), or "post-Covid syndrome."*

In the June 4, 2020, issue of *The Atlantic*, science writer Ed Yong writes that people belonging to support groups on Slack and Facebook "say they have been wrestling with serious Covid-19 symptoms for at least a month, if not two or three. Some call themselves 'long-termers' or 'long-haulers.'"

The term "long Covid" had been coined by Dr. Elisa Perego on May 20, 2020, as a Twitter hashtag to describe her own case of a persistent condition that differed greatly from the course of Covid assumed by most researchers. Long-haulers avoid euphemisms such as "post-Covid syndrome" because, as Perego writes in the *British Medical Journal (BMJ)* in October 2020, "we believe that to use 'chronic,' 'syndrome,' and 'post'" at present, when so little is known about cause(s) and mechanisms of long Covid, risks leaving those with long Covid behind, especially if and when an effective vaccine is distributed." Since then, effective vaccines have been distributed, and a great many people still suffer from long Covid. Figures from the CDC and the UK's Office for National Statistics suggest that one in ten Covid patients experience symptoms for twelve weeks or more.

Covid-19 normally lasts two weeks after the first symptoms, but longer-term, on-and-off symptoms— such as loss of taste and smell, a feeling of heaviness, general malaise, "brain fog," tight chest, and racing heart—persist in some patients for months. A neuro-scientist contacted by Yong was on her seventy-ninth day. Scottish journalist Vonny LeClerc told Yong that after suffering from severe symptoms for eighty days, she was still "reduced to not being able to stand up in the shower without feeling fatigued. I've tried going to the supermarket and I'm in bed for days afterwards. It's like nothing I've ever experienced before."

Early in the pandemic, Tim Spector, a genetics epidemiologist at King's College London, designed a Covid-19 tracker app to determine what proportion of the population was showing coronavirus symptoms; of the 4 million people who signed on to the app, 200,000 reported having symptoms that lasted for six weeks or longer. The app is operated by ZOE Global Limited, a nutrition advice company founded by Spector in

2017. Long-haulers going back to work while still feeling sick—and in one survey, 30 percent of health-care workers in Vancouver reported going to work at least once while feeling sick—became vectors for passing on the disease to others. "There is a whole other side to the virus which has not had attention," said Spector, "because of the idea that 'if you aren't dead you are fine.'"

The notion that Covid-19 was a short-term inconvenience was bolstered by people like Donald Trump, who assured Americans that the disease was "no worse than the flu," and that it was only the elderly and the weak who worried about it. The danger of that notion was that it lurked behind the concept of herd immunity, and gave credence to anti-mask and anti-vax protests. An anti-masker told a reporter at an airport in Arizona, "So I get Covid, so what? It's not like it's a serious disease." As Felicity Callard, a geographer at the University of Glasgow, put it, the misconception that Covid is mild and brief "establishes a framework in which 'not hiding' from the disease looks a manageable and sensible undertaking."

It's not unusual for patients with a severe disease to experience lingering symptoms after the disease has subsided, but long Covid affects even those who have had mild or even no symptoms. "It is notable," write Tae Chung et al., on the Johns Hopkins Medicine website, "that post-Covid-19 syndrome is not just afflicting people who were very sick with the coronavirus." Even asymptomatic patients find themselves suffering from long Covid, months after they didn't know they'd had the disease. Emily Pfeil Brigham, a pulmonologist at Johns Hopkins, noted that "patients who were never severely ill are coming to [the] clinic and saying that their lives are different now." Some studies do show, however, that patients showing five or more symptoms of Covid—fever, cough, fatigue, loss of taste or smell, brain fog, shortness of breath—in the early stages are more likely to develop long Covid.

Until recently, medical professionals have been telling long-haulers that they were making up their symptoms and that there is no such thing as long Covid, ignoring possibly significant similarities between long Covid and other illnesses with unexplained, lingering symptoms, such as chronic fatigue syndrome. But it's possible that that will change as evidence for long-term effects emerges with time. Some patients in China still have high levels of cardiac troponin, a marker for myocardial injury, long after their other Covid symptoms passed. The US Congress has given the NIH $1.15 billion for a project called the RECOVER Initiative (recovercovid.org), which is investigating long Covid. A significant proportion will go toward interviewing and treating long-haulers themselves. Long-haulers hope that soon they'll be able to emerge from behind a hashtag to get the full attention of the medical profession.

Uptick / *An economist's term for a small increase in a stock or commodity that has been steady or declining in the past. Applied to Covid, an increase in the number of daily reported cases, hospitalizations, or deaths.*

The ticker tape machine was invented in 1867 by Edward A. Calahan, an employee of the American Telegraph Company, when he placed a telegraph machine and operator on the floor of the New York Stock Exchange. The machine—called a ticker because of the noise made by the telegraph's type wheel—transmitted every change in the value of a stock as it was traded on the floor. Eventually, since every movement of a stock's value was recorded, every change was referred to as a "tick." An "uptick" occurred when a share's price rose in relation to its last tick, or trade. A "tick" was a small increase or decrease, not serious, nothing to make investors want to jump out of windows.

"World Health Organization Warns of Global Uptick in Covid Cases After Weeks of Decline," read the CNBC headline on March 3, 2021. That week, the world recorded 2.6 million new cases of Covid-19, an increase of 7 percent over the previous week, following six consecutive weeks of declines. Just an uptick, nothing to worry about.

On April 2, 2021, the *Montreal Gazette* noted that "Montreal's hospitals are beginning to report an uptick in Covid-19 admissions during the pandemic's third wave, with younger and sicker patients staying longer in intensive-care units." In Quebec, the number of new cases had "crept up" from 487 on April 1 to 503 on April 2.

"Though there may be an uptick of BA.2 infections in the coming months," write Prakash Nagarkatti and Mitzi Nagarkatti in The Conversation on March 22, 2022, "protective immunity from vaccination or previous infection provides defense against severe disease."

The word "uptick" is now being used in contexts where it almost certainly would not have been used before. In February 2021, for example, Ohio Common Pleas judge Eugene A. Lucci, in sentencing a man to prison for the illegal possession of a firearm, noted in his judgment that there had lately been "an uptick in interest by judges" in firearm safety training. During an American League Division Series baseball game in October 2021, a sportscaster commented that one of the Boston Red Sox players "would like to get his batting average up a tick." And in his 2021 book, *A Swim in a Pond in the Rain*, George Saunders notes that when our view of the main character in Anton Chekhov's short story "In the Cart" changes from that of a blameless victim to that of someone partially responsible for her own unhappiness, "the result is an uptick in our attentiveness." Two years before, it is unlikely any of these would have used the word "uptick." They would have said they'd seen an "increase," or that a batting average needed to "move up a notch," or there would have been a "sharpening" of our attention.

If, as Canadian poet Robert Bringhurst has argued, language represents the taming of thought, then the use of a word in a new way must represent a new thought, or a change in our old way of thinking. In normal times, when there is no war or pandemic, a single death is a significant event. The deaths of ten or fifty people in a bus accident or airplane crash are reported as a tragedy. But during a pandemic, describing multiple deaths as an "uptick" means that individual deaths have become insignificant. Death is only a real concern when it comes in "surges."

On October 27, 2021, the Associated Press reported that "overall, WHO's vast Americas region—which has tallied the most deaths of any region from the pandemic, at more than 2.7 million—saw a 1-percent uptick in deaths over the last week, even as cases fell by 9 percent." That day, twenty-one countries in the Americas recorded a combined total of 1,149 deaths. That is not an insignificant number of dead people. If 1,149 people had died at any other time, in any other kind of natural disaster—an earthquake in Haiti, a forest fire in California, a flood in Bangladesh—the world would have recoiled in shock and horror. But during the pandemic, when 1,149 people died in a single day, it was just an uptick, almost a positive thing. Hardly an increase at all. We were lucky it wasn't a surge.

Gene Drive / *The technique of genetically modifying an organism's genome with a new trait so that the organism will pass that trait on to its offspring—and potentially to all future descendants of that organism—thereby suddenly modifying the entire species.*

In June 2021, virologists Yaniv Erlich of Israel's Reichman University (formerly known as the Interdisciplinary Center Herzliya) and Daniel Douek of NIAID in the US proposed using gene drive to render horseshoe bats in China immune to coronaviruses. Since horseshoe bats are the suspected source of the coronavirus that caused Covid-19, Erlich and Douek thought that by rewriting the bats' DNA to resist infection, they would prevent future outbreaks of viral pandemics. The proposal has yet to be taken up by the scientific community.

As a technique, gene drive has been in use since 2011, when geneticists Austin Burt and Andrea Crisanti planted a gene in the genome of a laboratory population of mosquitoes; the genome radiated into 100 percent of the insects' descendants instead of into only half of them, as would have happened by the usual process of inherited characteristics. This was the first time that an altered gene had been inserted into an organism with the gene editing tool CRISPR, which caused the inserted gene to copy itself onto its partner chromosome so that the insect's genome no longer had the natural version—two different chromosomes, one from each parent—but instead had two copies of the altered gene, which was then passed on to all offspring.

As Anthony A. James, a biologist at the University of California, Irvine, explains, the technique has human applications. For example, gene drive could ensure that all future offspring of one brown-eyed parent and one blue-eyed parent would have blue eyes, and that the gene for blue eyes would become dominant in all descendants of the couple. The potential for genetically manipulating humans in other, less trivial ways, is both enthralling and frightening. Gene drive could ensure that no child of a parent suffering from a genetic disorder such as Huntington's disease would be born with that genetic possibility, but it could also ensure that every descendant of a racially mixed couple would have white skin.

In 2016, the National Academy of Sciences (NAS) cautiously recognized gene drive as a promising technological innovation that could, in a relatively short time, eliminate species that cause diseases in humans. For example, agriculturists in the US have experimented with gene drive modifications to the spotted wing fruit fly, a major pest for raspberries and blackberries. The NAS cautions, however, that several crucial questions need to be answered before gene drive can be approved for use outside a laboratory. Could the new trait jump from the modified species to another, closely related species? And, even more germane to the coronavirus issue, by eliminating one species of virus, could gene drive open the door for another, deadlier virus to take over the evolutionary niche?

Apart from the technical difficulties—gene drive has never been accomplished outside controlled laboratory conditions—the idea of altering the natural evolutionary process in a wild species, or eliminating an entire species, even if it is a species of virus that has killed at least 15 million humans in two years (some scientists suggest as many as 18.2 million people have died from Covid), gives bioethicists pause. Natalie Kofler, a molecular biologist and founder of Editing Nature, a bioethics organization that pushes for ethical considerations when making scientific decisions, urges that there are other, safer ways to reduce the risk of future pandemics. "We need to be thinking about changing the unhealthy relationship of humans and nature," she told STAT on July 1, 2021, "not to gene drive a wild animal so that we can continue our irresponsible and unsustainable behavior that is going to come back and bite us in the ass in the future."

Vaccine Passport / *A digital app or paper certificate verifying that a person has been fully vaccinated against Covid-19, or has recently tested negative for the virus, or has recovered from having Covid-19; required in some jurisdictions for access to restaurants, concerts, and international travel.*

On April 6, 2021, the *New York Times* reported that vaccine passports "are shaping up to be the next big clash in the American culture wars."

Not only in the US. Two months earlier, despite rising second-wave cases and slow vaccine rollouts throughout the European Union, member governments, fearful of losing a second tourism season, eased restrictions on restaurants and other tourist-related enterprises and called for the creation of digital documentation that would allow travel within the EU without a lot of paperwork and quarantining. On March 17, the governments submitted a proposal to the European Commission for something called a Digital Green Certificate (DGC), which would be valid in all EU countries. They were also working with the World Health Organization to see if the DGC could be recognized worldwide.

With most of its population vaccinated and Covid cases down by 90 percent, Israel announced in February 2021 that it would issue a "Green Pass" phone app to citizens one week after their second shot, granting access to bars, restaurants, hotels, and recreational facilities such as gyms and swimming pools. Greece, Cyprus, and Georgia said they would recognize Israel's Green Pass.

In March, China issued a digital vaccine passport that ran on Tencent's WeChat phone app, which could be scanned for access to buses and stores.

But resistance to vaccine passports soon surfaced. Arguments against them were ethical, practical, and legal. In the US, in April 2021, when only 19 percent of the American population had been vaccinated, the debate was whether institutions like schools could legally require such passports; if so, that would be the equivalent of mandating vaccinations, which some felt to be unconstitutional. Some states, such as Texas, Florida, Pennsylvania, and Arkansas, drafted legislation that banned or limited the issuing or requiring of vaccine passports, claiming that such documents were socialist intrusions on an individual's right to make private health choices.

An argument in favor of digital documentation was that it would be more difficult to fake a digital app than it had been to buy false "proofs" of negative Covid tests, as several travelers coming from France were caught doing, or changing the dates on negative tests to get past health checks, as happened in Brazil and Canada. In February 2021, just before the announcement of the EU's DGC, the European law enforcement agency Europol notified border control officers that a man had been arrested in London Luton Airport trying to sell false coronavirus test results to travelers. And in January 2022, unvaccinated Serbian tennis pro Novak Djokovic told Australian authorities that he had tested positive for Covid in Serbia in December and therefore was immune to the disease; some officials think he may have lied about the test. Having a phone app that could be scanned at airports would make such issues a lot clearer.

The objection in Canada was that because there was no solid evidence that vaccination made a person noninfectious, issuing vaccine passports might allow infectious persons to mingle with the general population. There was also the worry that vaccine passports would create a two-tiered situation within a country, with some citizens allowed to travel and others not— for example, in Canada, a person aged sixty-four years would have been vaccinated months before someone who was twenty-five, and therefore would be allowed to travel much sooner. Similarly, countries that could afford to have a high proportion of their citizens vaccinated would have an advantage over those that could not. As Lori Turnbull, director of Dalhousie University's School of Public Administration, told CTV News on March 9, 2021, "if we see some parts of the world that are not able to get into this conversation because they don't have access to vaccines, that's a global problem."

Canada relented in September 2021, however, when the majority of Canadians were vaccinated and ready to travel, and the US, the UK, and many European countries said they would refuse entry to anyone without proof of being fully vaccinated. The push came from the major airlines, who complained that requiring paper proof of vaccination of the kind then being issued by Health Canada was not enough; they wanted a government-issued, digitized passport that could be quickly scanned at boarding gates and would be recognized abroad. As of October 30, 2021, all passengers boarding domestic or international flights in Canada needed to show vaccine passports, which were provided by their provinces. That requirement was lifted on March 1, 2022.

How readily passports were accepted may have depended on how authorities described their purpose. An article on The Conversation in September 2021 suggested that the way a question is "framed" to the public determines how it is answered. For example, in European countries, where there were few restrictions and lockdowns, people who were vaccinated worried about being infected by anti-vaxxers. There, the question of whether or not to issue "Green Passes" was framed to imply that because vaccine passports restricted the freedom of the unvaccinated, going into a restaurant or getting on a train or airplane would be safer if everyone was required to show a Green Pass.

In Australia, however, where there were heavy restrictions, frequent lockdowns, and closed borders for long stretches of time, the question was framed differently: a vaccine passport would give bearers more freedom to enter bars and restaurants and to travel, allowing them to return to a semblance of normal life. It was a matter of language. A vaccine passport offered both restrictions to the unvaccinated and freedom to the vaccinated, but how the case was put to the public determined how voters responded to the question.

Languishing / *The sense of purposelessness or stagnation felt by some during the second year of the pandemic. Defined by sociologists as the absence of well-being.*

Adam Grant, in the *New York Times* on April 19, 2021, calls this sense of emptiness "the dominant emotion of 2021." He writes, "It wasn't burnout—we still had energy. It wasn't depression—we didn't feel hopeless. We just felt somewhat joyless and aimless."

The term "languishing" was coined by sociologist Corey Keyes in his 2002 journal article "The Mental Health Continuum: From Languishing to Flourishing in Life." Keyes identified the feeling as existing somewhere between depression and flourishing, but closer to depression. In fact, he said, languishing is "the prelude to depression." It's a form of grief; after two years of lockdowns and putting our lives on hold, we are mourning the loss of normalcy.

The pandemic has been traumatic for a great many people. Studies in Italy have found that those who described themselves as languishing in 2020 were three times as likely as those who did not describe themselves that way to be diagnosed with post-traumatic stress disorder in 2021.

6

The After Times

"Actually, I don't exactly have expectations. I have hopes, and fears. Mostly, the fears predominate."

URSULA K. LE GUIN

"They used to ask me all kinds of questions:
Will I get a good husband
Will I be rich
Will the baby recover
and so on.
Now it's only the one thing:
Is there no hope?"

MARGARET ATWOOD, "Another Visit to the Oracle"

Breakthrough Infection / *A case of Covid-19 in a person fourteen or more days after that person has received all recommended doses of an authorized Covid-19 vaccine.*

Some people who have been fully vaccinated against a particular disease may still contract the disease: getting a flu shot doesn't necessarily mean you won't get the flu. Flu vaccines are 58 percent effective, but studies show that being vaccinated against the flu reduces the risk of illness by between 40 and 50 percent among the general population. Although some vaccines against Covid-19 are 94 percent effective, there is still a small risk of illness among vaccinated persons. A certain number of breakthrough infections are anticipated.

Apart from chance, post-vaccine infections can be caused by inadequate storage of the vaccine, mutations in the virus that render the vaccine less effective (during surges of the Alpha, Delta, and Omicron variants, breakthrough infections also surged), biological factors such as patient age (people over sixty-five seem to be more susceptible), or the deterioration of memory B cells in the patient that are supposed to recognize and attack the invading virus. There is also some evidence of waning immunity, in which the effectiveness of vaccines declines a few months after immunization.

As of April 2021, 112 million Americans had been fully vaccinated, and 10,262 of them, about 0.009 percent, had had breakthrough infections. A study of double-vaccinated health-care workers at the Sheba Medical Center in Israel found that of the 1,497 workers tested, 37 of them, or about 2.5 percent, tested positive. The percentage was also low in Canada: breakthrough infections among fully vaccinated Canadians in June 2021 amounted to just 0.5 percent of the

Covid cases. By May, the CDC in the US had stopped tallying mild breakthrough infections, monitoring only severe cases; by then, 159 million people had been fully vaccinated, and 5,492 of them had been hospitalized and/or died. Of those, the majority (4,109 people) were sixty-five years old or older.

Still, as Katherine J. Wu writes in *The Atlantic* (July 13, 2021), the media has been "really, really bad at communicating" the fact that breakthroughs are expected and mild. A breakthrough infection, she writes, is "a concept that has, not entirely accurately, become synonymous with vaccine failure." As if to prove her point, an article on NBC News a few days later began, "Despite the power of Covid-19 vaccines in cutting the risk of hospitalization and death from the disease, fully vaccinated people can get very sick and die from the virus in rare cases." It is an axiom of journalism, apparently, that no news story can emphasize the positive; you will never read in a newspaper that of 159 million people vaccinated, 158,994,508 of them did not subsequently get severe Covid.

When dealing with the continuing presence of Covid in our lives, far more concerning than breakthrough infections is the number of Covid-19 cases that occur among the unvaccinated. A report released by the Ontario COVID-19 Science Advisory Table at the end of September 2021 stated that unvaccinated people were seven times as likely as vaccinated people to contract Covid-19, twenty-five times as likely to require hospitalization, and sixty times as likely to end up in an ICU. A similar study in King County, Washington, showed that from July to the end of August 2021, Covid cases among the unvaccinated increased from eight cases a day per 100,000 population to eighty-three cases a day, whereas in vaccinated persons the increase was from one case a day to nine a day. The same held true elsewhere—in Switzerland, at the height of the Omicron wave, deaths among the unvaccinated were 14.52 per 100,000; among the fully vaccinated, they were 1.41. In England, the figures were 23.8 and 5.2, respectively.

According to the WHO, there were 15 million new cases of Covid reported worldwide during the first week of January 2022, with about 50,000 deaths; "the overwhelming majority" of hospitalized cases were unvaccinated.

It was the prevalence of breakthrough infections that convinced many governments to make third, or booster, vaccine doses available, at first to vulnerable populations and then, with the advent of Omicron, to all citizens. Israel was the first to offer boosters, making third shots available to the elderly in July 2021, and to all citizens over twelve in August. Hungary also urged booster shots in August when studies showed that Sinopharm, the Chinese vaccine the country was using, "did not offer robust protection to the elderly," reported the *Washington Post*. The rest of the EU followed suit from October to mid-December. Despite ethical concerns about giving healthy people third shots (Israel began giving fourth shots in January 2022) when many in poorer countries had not received their first, after Omicron struck in the fall of 2022, thirty-six countries around the world were offering, and in some cases mandating, booster shots to protect against breakthrough infections.

Covexit; Pandexit / *The process of gradually easing and finally removing restrictions on public life mandated by health authorities in response to the pandemic.*

After an online "Construction Breakfast" held in April 2020 by Gregg Latchams, one of the oldest business consultancies in England, the firm reported that "construction contracts, employment matters and financial and business planning were all hot topics with our expert panel crystallising the story so far and what comes next as we move towards 'Covexit.'" The term "Covexit" was adapted from "Brexit," the withdrawal of the UK from the European Union that was to take place at midnight, December 31, 2020, suggesting that ending the pandemic would be as traumatic for everyone as withdrawing from the European Union was for Britain.

Perhaps the law firm was discussing a Covexit strategy because earlier that month the European Commission and the European Council had drawn up a joint European roadmap for eventually lifting the restrictions imposed on EU communities in response to the pandemic. They identified three prerequisites for a Covexit: clear scientific data, sufficient health-care system capacity, and appropriate monitoring ability. Over the next few weeks, as more cases of Covid were reported, more criteria were added in antici-pation of a possible second wave precipitated by the relaxing of restrictions. Among the new criteria were proof of a sustained and consistent decline in new cases and deaths, the ability to conduct widespread testing, and enough medical equipment to meet a new spike in infections. Any withdrawal of restrictions before those conditions were met would lead to wide-spread political, medical, and economic disaster.

In many countries, however, economic pressures forced governments to relax restrictions within weeks of putting them into effect—with predicted results. On May 20, 2020, the *New York Times* reported that some schools in France had to be closed again only a week after reopening because of spikes in new cases, and in Iran, weeks after the easing of restrictions in April, the number of new cases rose in eight provinces. "Health experts attributed the resurgence to the coun-try's reopening before cases were consistently falling," reported the *Times*, "and before Iran had established widespread testing and contact tracing."

On April 18, Adam Radwanski and Ivan Semeniuk, writers for the *Globe and Mail*, asked, "What Will

Canada's Pandexit Strategy Look Like?" They warned that Canadians "should be braced for a potentially frustrating and anxiety-inducing second phase of the coronavirus response," as provinces and the federal government met to work out their own roadmap to putting a too-early end to restrictions.

That May, "Covexit" was a Collins Dictionary "new word suggestion." The dictionary cited a prescient article from the *British Medical Journal (BMJ)* that stated, "Covexit will not remain confined to the hospital setting. We should expect a long and exhausting fight that will involve all health-care workers, citizens' compliance and international collaboration."

Although the three conditions for a smooth Pandexit identified by the joint European roadmap in April 2020 were never completely met, most countries began lifting restrictions anyway, with the result that populations were hit with successive waves of new infections. When it came to a choice of "lives or livelihoods," governments around the world consistently chose livelihoods. The few exceptions—Australia, New Zealand, Iceland—were regarded dubiously, almost with a kind of pity, certainly not emulated, even though their Covid numbers at the time were astonishingly low (those countries, too, eventually lifted restrictions, and their numbers rose accordingly). Former New Jersey governor Chris Christie—defending the White House decision to reopen businesses in the US in May 2020, when 70,000 people had already died and the number of new cases was climbing daily—put the case succinctly: "Of course, everybody wants to save every life they can," he told CNN, "but the question is, towards what end?"

By March 2021, as a third wave of Covid-19 cases swept the world, it was clear that any Pandexit was going to be a rocky road. Writing in a working paper for BIS, the Bank for International Settlements (a forum for the world's central banks based in Basel, Switzerland), Phurichai Rungcharoenkitkul comments that "unexpected setbacks could still disrupt the 'pandexit.'" The pace of vaccination rollouts could be slow, virus mutations could proliferate, and governments could respond too hastily to apparent decreases in new cases. All three setbacks occurred simultaneously: a perfect storm of new cases, massive hospitalizations, and Covid deaths. At the time, the economic impact of the pandemic was a median loss to the world's top twenty-seven economies of 2.25 percent. If a fourth wave followed the third (and it did), Rungcharoenkitkul calculated that the output loss could go to 3 or 3.75 percent; if new variants appeared that resulted in loss of immunity (and they did), then the impact would rise to an output loss of 5 percent in 2021. When all of those conditions arose, Rungcharoenkitkul's worst-case scenario was realized.

BIS general manager Agustín Carstens said that as the pandemic receded, economies would need to be slowly weaned off the life-support payments they had received from central banks to avoid a run of corporate insolvencies. And since house prices had risen far more than expected during Covid, that sector would be more vulnerable than usual if interest rates rose significantly after the pandemic was over and people were unable to make the high interest payments. As a result, a recession such as was seen in the US in 2008 could recur. Carstens emphasized the need for banks to keep interest rates low, but despite his appeals, by June 2021 the central banks of six countries—Russia, Turkey, Brazil, the Czech Republic, Hungary, and Mexico—had raised their rates.

In Canada, the Bank of Canada was expected to raise its prime interest rate from 2.45 percent to 3.45 percent by the end of 2022. "The 1-percent difference," reports the *Queens Citizen*, "will cause [variable] mortgage rates to increase by over 40 percent. This will drastically affect the borrowers of variable-rate mortgages." By June 2022, the prime rate had been raised to 3.7 percent. The fixed mortgage rate was expected to increase from 4.74 percent to 6.95 percent by the end of 2024, a 46 percent increase in three years.

In a blog post published by *Forbes* on July 1, 2021, Cindy Gordon reported that the current estimate for the loss to the global economy in 2020 was 4.5 percent. "To put this number in perspective," she writes, "global GDP was estimated at around 87.55 trillion US dollars in 2019—meaning that a 4.5 percent drop in economic growth results in almost 3.94 trillion US dollars of lost economic output." Current estimates for global GDP losses in 2021 are 5.6 percent.

For many, the economic situation after Covexit could be as severe as it was during Covid.

Freedom Day / *July 19, 2021; the day British prime minister Boris Johnson arbitrarily lifted most Covid restrictions in the UK, allowing the reopening of bars, restaurants, and workplaces, removing all limits on outdoor gatherings, and marking the end of mandatory masking and social distancing.*

Johnson's original date for Freedom Day had been June 21, 2021, but the emancipation was postponed for four weeks because of a spike in cases caused by the Delta variant. At the time, only 53 percent of the British population had been fully vaccinated.

Two days before the new Freedom Day, 54,000 new Covid cases were recorded in the UK, and health authorities urged Johnson to delay the reopening again, or even to cancel it. Many regional political leaders said they would override the government, at least on the issue of face masks, by insisting that masks and social distancing continue on public transport. Andy Burnham, the mayor of Greater Manchester, warned that "Freedom Day" would in fact be "Anxiety Day" for huge numbers of vulnerable people—the elderly, the

unvaccinated, those with respiratory weaknesses—
who had to travel on buses, trollies, and trains.

But Johnson—who was himself in quarantine
because he'd been in contact with his health secretary, Sajid Javid, who'd tested positive for Covid on July
17—refused to back down. He did, however, say that he
expected Britons to behave responsibly—to continue
wearing face masks and to maintain social distance—
and two-thirds of the population said they intended
to do so.

But the other third partied as if there were no
tomorrow.

On the morning of July 22, following the joyous
reopening of pubs and nightclubs, thousands of people who were allowed to return to work chose not to,
because the NHS Covid-19 track-and-trace apps on
their cell phones had pinged, warning them that the
night before—Freedom Night—they had been in close
contact with someone who had tested positive, and
advising them to self-isolate for ten days. Or so they
said. The resulting disruption to the country's factories, railways, supermarkets, and schools, which were
all supposed to have been open and fully staffed, was
dubbed a "pingdemic."

Later that day, the British government announced
that fully vaccinated workers in critical roles—air traffic controllers and train signalers, for example—could
return to work despite having been pinged.

Two weeks later, British health authorities were predicting that as a result of the unlocking, new cases in the UK would soar to more than 100,000 a day. As the online publication The Naked Scientists reported on July 30, "over 100 scientists signed a letter to the *Lancet* medical journal, stating 'the Government is embarking on a dangerous and unethical experiment, and we call on it to pause plans to abandon mitigation.'"

Predicting 100,000 new cases was probably a mistake; by the end of August, new cases in the UK were at 30,000 a day—still high, but seeming low because it wasn't 100,000. Hospital admissions were rising at the rate of 6.7 percent a week and deaths were averaging 133 a day, and yet people partied on. The last week in August, 60,000 soccer fans crowded into Emirates Stadium to watch a match between Arsenal and Chelsea, and Andrew Lloyd Webber's musical *Cinderella* debuted in London. The *New York Times* noted that the London Underground was packed with passengers, and although face masks on public transit were again mandated, only half the travelers wore them. "We don't seem to care that we have these really high infection rates," epidemiologist Tim Spector told the *Times*. "It looks like we're just accepting it now—that this is the price of freedom."

Great Resignation / *The wave of employee resigna-tions that occurred after Covid restrictions were lifted in 2021, when people who had been working at home for a year and a half decided they didn't want to go back to their old jobs. Also called the "Big Quit."*

According to a survey of 30,000 employees conducted by the US Department of Labor in April 2021, 41 per-cent of people who had been working at home said they were considering quitting or changing their jobs when the pandemic was over. That month, 7 percent of them did quit, a jump over the ten-year quit rate of 2–3 percent. The rise prompted Texas A&M busi-ness professor Anthony Klotz to predict that the year would see a "Great Resignation" as people continued to redefine their attitudes toward the traditional nine-to-five routine. Klotz proved to be right. In July, 4.4 million more Americans handed in their pink slips. That month, *Forbes* reported that one in three employ-ees said they would quit their jobs if they could no longer work from home.

In Canada, the number of employees who quit their jobs in June 2021 was triple the number of those who had quit in the same month in 2020. And it wasn't just entry-level employees—junior clerks and restau-rant waitpersons—who were quitting. Half the senior managers surveyed by RBC Economics said they were considering retiring or stepping down to less demanding roles. The mass exodus affected all types of employment, but the professional, scientific, and technical fields were hit hardest. In those areas, there was a 4.6 percent vacancy rate, compared with 3.6 percent across all job fronts. As Derek Thompson writes in *The Atlantic* in October 2021, "That Great Resignation? It just keeps getting greater."

Thompson attributed the mass exodus to several tangible factors: pandemic relief checks, rent moratoriums, and the forgiving of student loans. With so many government-sponsored safety nets, people didn't have to go back to work. Holly Corbett, writing in *Forbes*, sees other causes for the Great Resignation—pandemic burnout, for example—and also noted that for many workers, going back to the office meant returning to cubicles, being unable to walk the dog or play with the kids, worrying about what to wear, and a host of other minor factors that added up to a decision to say no. As Dr. LaNail R. Plummer, a psychologist with the Onyx Therapy Group, put it, the pandemic gave many people a year and a half in which to make the "decision to prioritize self."

For many workers, though, working from home meant spending less money on clothes, restaurant lunches, and parking, less time commuting to and from the workplace, more time with the family (not sending the children to day care, because there was no day care), and more time working when they felt most creative, which might have been after the kids went to bed. Some didn't want to go back to a workplace where racist, ageist, or sexist discrimination poisoned the atmosphere. Others realized during the pandemic that they just didn't like where they were working and wanted to explore other opportunities. Still others, after a year and a half of feeling safe in semi-isolation, were reluctant to go back to working in a crowded office with other people who may or may not have been vaccinated.

Derek Thompson sees the Great Resignation as a positive thing, an indication that people may be taking the opportunity to exercise more control over their lives. "Quitting," he writes, "is really an expression of optimism that says, 'We can do better.'" Even those who kept their jobs while working from home found time to develop other pursuits. A woman I know took up photography; another studied jazz piano. Another moved in with her mother and took online courses in eldercare. More women were quitting than men. In August 2021, when another 4.4 million American workers quit their jobs, the number of women who quit was 1.1 percentage points higher than it was for men.

Taking up new pursuits is the kind of thing people do when they retire, and it may be that the pandemic has been, for many people, a kind of retirement, in which work receded from the foreground and was replaced by actual living. In French, "retirement" is *retraite*, more like a retreat, a stepping away; perhaps, psychologically, we have been in retreat—almost in a religious sense—for two years, in which we have withdrawn from the world and now are reluctant to plunge back into it. As Thompson points out, the "quitters" may in fact be part of a growing movement that refuses to put work at the center of their lives. "We may... look back to the pandemic," he writes, "as a crucial inflection point in something more fundamental" than a simple dissatisfaction with office politics and long commutes. We may be experiencing a profound shift in our attitudes toward work.

Cave Syndrome / *An unwillingness to leave the comfort and safety of home, even after the pandemic abates and restrictions are lifted; a lingering fear of infection or discomfort in social situations. An extension of coronaphobia.*

I knew a man who suffered from agoraphobia so extreme that he left his apartment only once during the twenty years of our acquaintance. He rarely allowed anyone to visit him. Friends or family members would buy his groceries and leave them in the hallway outside his door with his mail. He died several days before he was found. In Japan, agoraphobia that profound is called *hikikomori*, which translates as "turning inward" and is usually brought on by early childhood trauma.

Cave syndrome is similar to *hikikomori* but is brought on by prolonged isolation during the pandemic and, notwithstanding the age of my friend, is particularly prevalent in young people and adolescents, writes Ravi Chandra in *Psychology Today*, adding that "the traumatized and anxious are important bellwethers of our society." People with cave syndrome, then, are the hidden, fragile canaries that tell us we are not allowing enough air into the mine shaft. Experiences that most of us accept as part of everyday living—as "the price of freedom"—are, for some, deeply disturbing disruptions in the present that connect subconsciously with deeply disturbing disruptions in the past.

Arthur Bregman, a Florida psychiatrist, coined the term "cave syndrome" in March 2021 to describe "the isolation you crave" even when staying home is no longer mandated by health authorities. "A lot of people are scared to death of going out," he said. "People can't shake the anxiety. They feel fearful and insecure about the uncertainty of the situation." Cave syndrome is a milder form of agoraphobia than my friend exhibited—being reluctant to go shopping is different from being terrified of leaving the house—but it's still an indication that the pandemic has been a traumatic experience for all of us, however much we think we are shaking it off. The phrase is new, but the syndrome itself is very old.

George Bonanno, a clinical psychologist at Columbia University who studies the effects of hurricanes, terrorist attacks, and widespread traumas such as the 2003 SARS outbreak, says there are three common responses to traumatic events: 65 percent of people remain relatively unaffected after the trauma, 25 percent experience temporary depression or stress disorders, and 10 percent suffer from long-lasting psychological debilities.

The transition from isolation back into society, writes Anna Russell in the *New Yorker* (June 3, 2021), can be "a little bumpy." She cites a survey conducted by the American Psychological Association, which found that 49 percent of adult Americans reported anticipating that they will feel "uneasy about adjusting to in-person interaction once the pandemic ends"—especially the kind of in-person interactions that involve crowded, enclosed areas, such as airplanes, buses, trains, movie theaters, workplaces, and restaurants. For them, the pandemic has been "a transformational experience." For one of us in ten, coping with reentry after the pandemic will produce symptoms identical to those that appear after major disasters.

Cave syndrome appears in a number of guises. Another person I know wears a face mask to bed at night; another continues to shop online even though the stores have reopened. One out of ten of us does not want to leave our home. In the final scene of *Inside*, American comedian Bo Burnham's selfie-documentary of the year he spent shut up in his home, Burnham hesitantly leaves his house, loses his nerve, and ends up pounding on the door to get back in. Some of us will simply find the prospect of working in an office, eating in a crowded restaurant, or commuting on a bus too risky. Statistics Canada estimates that tourism revenue in Canada fell by 50 percent in 2020 and predicted it would take five years to return to normal; in other words, for many of us, returning to our previous ways of living will be a gradual process, and some of us won't return at all.

Revenge Travel / *A surge in tourism as the number of Covid cases declines and airlines and cruise ships reopen, which some feel redresses the injustice of travel restrictions imposed during the pandemic. The opposite of cave syndrome.*

A headline in the *Washington Post* on July 29, 2020, reads: " 'Revenge Travel' Is the Phenomenon That Could Bring Back Tourism With a Bang." The hope expressed was that after a long period of suppressed travel because of pandemic restrictions, when tourism revenue in some countries dried up, people would travel even more when the crisis was over. "A sense of wanderlust has been building," writes Caroline Bologna in HuffPost. "It's only natural that we'll want to explore new places after so much time at home."

In Europe, according to the European Travel Commission, where many borders remained closed to nonessential traffic as Covid cases continued to mount despite vaccinations, "data to January [2021] indicates an 85 percent plunge in international tourist arrivals... and travel demand is now expected to remain below its pre-pandemic trajectory until 2024." But domestic travel returned with greater vengeance, and revenues in the first quarter of 2022 were up 280 percent over 2021 levels in Europe, 117 percent in the Americas, and 132 percent in the Middle East, even though the total number of travelers was well below 2019 levels.

"Post-pandemic travel," according to Chris Choi, a professor of hospitality, food, and tourism management at the University of Guelph, "will be in great demand. It's called the 'revenge travel' phenomenon. The problem is that it's going to be expensive." Post-pandemic travel might be all right, but when will we be post-pandemic? Choi, quoted in the July/August 2021 issue of *The Walrus*, found that hotels and vacation sites near large cities were fully booked in June 2021, which decidedly was not post-pandemic, and that prices were much higher than they had been before the pandemic. People were willing to spend money they'd saved by staying home. "This is going to be the reality for the next two years," said Choi.

Compared with travel recovery after SARS, which took fifteen years to return to pre-pandemic levels, two to three years would be a very quick bounce back. Perhaps too quick. That we are keen to travel when travel becomes safe again is understandable—but when is "safe," and where does the "revenge" come in? Revenge against the places we were not allowed to visit during the pandemic? Or revenge against the pandemic itself?

It's the latter, according to Eric Jones, cofounder of the website The Vacationer, who says that "the term is also retribution against Covid-19 and how it is losing its power to control our lives, including canceling travel plans." But lifting restrictions on travel, like ending restrictions on restaurants and beaches, is dangerous if undertaken too soon. Could revenge travel be a result of Covid-19's making us want to socialize, to go out and spread the virus? Could revenge travel be Covid's revenge on us for trying to snuff it out?

Jumping the gun seemed to raise the notion that we have a right to travel and that that right was denied us by Covid. "Revenge travel," writes Pete McMartin in the *Vancouver Sun*, is "a term that contained the air of self-entitlement and presumption that characterizes our appetite for travel." Such a notion ties "revenge travel" with "overtourism," the pushing of our inalienable right to travel to the point of ever-increasing carbon levels, accelerating species decline, more frequent contact with virus-bearing wild animals (and other human beings), and a degree of globalization that reduces the cultural differences between home and away. "You fly to a foreign city to experience life different from your own," says McMartin, "and find, instead, a Gap."

Merilyn and I returned to Mexico in October 2021, when travel seemed safe even though Covid lingered in the air. Live audience indoor performances were still banned, the cultural center and the opera house were closed, and some of the restaurants and cafés we had frequented before Covid—places that in Mexico are ephemeral at the best of times—were gone. Those that remained posted greeters at the door who sprayed our hands with disinfectant and took our temperatures with a kind of digitized ray gun that beeped and said, "*Temperatura normal.*" The places that were open catered to expats and tourists from Mexico City, known in San Miguel as *chilangos*, which didn't seem to make anyone happy. San Miguel felt like an occupied city.

Our friend, the Mexican poet Pedro Serrano, had written to us from Mexico City in May, warning that the capital, indeed the entire country, was in a state of confusion and turmoil. Enduring the pandemic, he wrote, felt as though "we all entered into this long tunnel of uncertain walls." He added, "I suppose that's what sailors experienced during those long expeditions to discover remote parts of the world. Now remoteness is happening every day in a tiny corner of everybody's room."

It appears that we want to travel to escape from our own remoteness.

Endemicity / *The post-pandemic future in which Covid-19 has become endemic—not eradicated but simple, accepted, and predictable.*

Hassan Vally and Catherine Bennett, writing for The Conversation on January 31, 2022, define "endemic" as a stage in a widespread infection when "we start to live alongside the virus." Life after a pandemic or epidemic returns to normal, except that one more pathogen has been added to the list of diseases we hear about and sometimes get. Few epidemiologists see that as a good thing. As Oxford virus evolutionist Aris Katzourakis writes in *Nature* (January 24, 2022), "the word 'endemic' has become one of the most misused of the pandemic."

Jacob Stern and Katherine J. Wu, in *The Atlantic*, call this stage "endemicity." And it worries them, because it is too closely associated with complacency. When a disease becomes endemic, we stop thinking about it as a disease and start thinking of it as an inconvenience, "no more concerning than a flu or common cold." Or even as a good thing, an excuse to stay home from work to read a good book.

The truth is, they write, "endemicity promises exactly none of this." For one thing, influenza *is* concerning to a great many people. The WHO estimates that, worldwide, somewhere between 290,000 and 650,000 people die of it every year. And not just in lower-income countries—about 28,000 people a year die of the flu in the US, and 8,000 in Canada. "Endemicity, then, just identifies a pathogen that's fixed itself in our population so stubbornly that we cease to be seriously perturbed by it. We tolerate it." Often to our cost.

Because the other problem with endemicity is that there is no guarantee that if it does come, it will be as mild as the flu. There are many ways in which a disease can become endemic, and not all of them are ways we'd be content to live with. HIV/AIDS is an endemic disease, as are malaria (600,000 deaths in 2020) and tuberculosis (1.5 million deaths in 2020).

"It is an unfortunate coincidence," write Stern and Wu, "that the word *endemic* begins with *end*." Endemicity is not the end, they say. "The arrival of endemicity is actually the beginning."

After Times / *A time, perpetually in the future, when the Covid-19 pandemic will be over.*

In March 2021, in a piece about restaurants in the US that had made it through the first year of Covid by making innovative pivots, the *New York Times* noted that establishments "that survived the pandemic—or even opened in the midst of it—may carry their adaptations into the After Times."

Note that the *Times* did not say "when things return to normal." Restaurants selling flowers and frozen lasagna is not normal. "Normal is never coming back,"

Laurie Penny writes on Medium. And she is right. When a forest burns or is cut down, it grows back, but the new forest is not the same as the old one. It has not only new trees but also new species of trees; new animals have moved in—birds hitherto unknown to it nest in its branches, and they will feed on new seeds and new insects. "Instead of remembering lasts," Penny adds, "we will start counting firsts."

The term "aftertime" appeared in English in 1557, when it simply meant "later," sometime after the events under discussion had taken place. In *Henry IV, Part 2*, Lord Hastings predicts that the uprising against King Henry will persist far into the future, from father to son, "whiles England shall have generation." Prince John, Henry's son, rebukes him, "You are too shallow, Hastings, much too shallow, / To sound the bottom of the after-times."

We are all too shallow to predict the future, but that hasn't stopped us from prognosticating about the post-pandemic world. Most forecasters foresee an increase in employees working from home (so common it is shortened to WFH) rather than returning to an office (RTO)—online companies such as Unilever, Continuum Global Solutions, and Culdesac have already announced that they are reducing their brick-and-mortar operations to let more, if not most, workers work remotely when the crisis is over. Culdesac closed its San Francisco offices and moved entirely online, and in May 2020 Shopify declared itself a "digital by default company" until the pandemic ends, "and after that, most [employees] will permanently work remotely."

This trend caused *The Economist* to predict a huge amount of untenanted office space. "Even small drops in occupancy rates," it pointed out, "will have a big effect on rents and prices," noting that the International Monetary Fund estimated that "a rise in vacancy rates of five percentage points in all commercial property would cause valuations to fall by 15 percent over five years." In the US, Moody's Investors Service, a rating agency, predicted that one-fifth of the country's offices would be empty by 2022.

Other predictions included more online shopping, which would mean more work for delivery services like FedEx and more dependence on payment by credit card and apps like PayPal. This in turn will lead more quickly to the cashless society that wasn't expected to arrive for another decade, as people decline to return to shopping in crowded malls and become more comfortable giving financial information online. In 2021, cash payments in the UK dropped by 35 percent. In Sweden, so many customers made their payments using a transfer service called Swish that "to swish" became a verb, much as "to debit," "to Venmo," and "to e-Transfer" are verbs in the US and Canada.

In many cities, parking meters can be fed using a smartphone app; more of that will happen. Restaurants will continue to put their menus and take-out orders on a phone app that is activated at the table by a

QR code. Even before the end of Covid, we were paying for theater tickets and choosing seats online. The farmers at our farmers market, who before Covid took only cash at their stalls, now take credit cards. I've seen customers use debit or credit cards for a two-dollar purchase at a supermarket, or to pay for a coffee at Tim Hortons. Even small retail outlets issue loyalty cards to customers; we're all going to need bigger wallets with more slots for all those cards. Cash is viewed with surprise, or even suspicion—who has touched this money? In the US and the UK, forensic scientists say that 80 to 90 percent of banknotes carry trace amounts of cocaine, which means that one end of almost every bill in your wallet has been in someone's nose.

There are downsides to going cashless, of course, and we will experience all of them. To use a transfer service, you have to have a smartphone and a bank account, meaning you have to have two pieces of identification from a list that includes a valid driver's license, passport, birth certificate, or other forms of government documentation—and this will screen out the poor and the homeless as much as it irks members of far-right vigilante groups. And then, every purchase made with a smartphone is traceable; someone somewhere could be taking note of it. Also, banks and computers are not infallible. Unless you're playing Monopoly, bank errors are seldom in the client's favor, and things often fall apart.

In August 2021, we were in a restaurant—seated inside, for the first time in months—when there was a power outage. The whole city went black. For two weeks, we had been caught in a massive heat wave, and the increased use of air conditioners had caused a brownout. Using the flashlight function on her cell phone, our waiter tallied our bill by hand, with a pencil and paper, but couldn't take our credit card because, hello, there was no internet. She offered to write down our credit card information and enter it later, when the power came back on, but I had a more secure solution: I paid with cash. Few others in the restaurant were able to do so.

But the more worrisome aspects of the After Times are the potential long-term psychological effects, especially on those who contracted Covid-19 and never fully recovered from it. Lingering malaises may include not only anxiety and depression but also the physical problems associated with those conditions, such as fatigue, sleep disorders, brain fog, and "a general sense of not being at your best," says Teodor Postolache, a psychologist at the University of Maryland School of Medicine. According to Postolache, "between 30 and 50 percent of people with [a coronavirus] infection that has clinical manifestations are going to have some form of mental health issues." Wes Ely, a critical care physician at Vanderbilt University Medical Center, believes that what started as a temporary reaction to being ill will become for some "a chronic illness" that manifests as numb limbs, headache, dizziness, and continued loss of smell and taste.

Those who did not contract Covid-19 but who worried that they would are also at risk of long-term negative effects. "Ongoing uncertainty takes a big toll," says Karestan Koenen, a Harvard professor of psychiatric epidemiology. "That's the basis of a traumatic stressor—unpredictability, uncontrollability—until it exceeds the ability of the organism to cope." As if in corroboration, *Harper's Magazine* reported in its April 2021 issue the results of a poll that found that 62 percent of American adults "believe that the pandemic has meaningfully damaged their mental health."

In Mexico there's a word for people who have survived a disaster: *damnificados*. The damaged ones. Or perhaps the damned. Virginia Simonds, a psychologist in Ottawa who has been treating depression and anxiety for years, says that "the difference between previous causes of these conditions and this pandemic is the insidiousness of it. It affects all aspects of our lives. Whereas before a client may have felt depressed about her job, or her family, something specific, now she's depressed about everything. It's as though the whole world is off its axis."

Traditionally, when the world is off its axis, major changes take place, some positive, some not so much. Historians have noted that deep, permanent, political, social, and cultural changes follow major disasters.

After the devastation of the Black Death, which, in the fourteenth century, killed roughly half the population of Europe—mostly members of the working and peasant classes—the new normal included the rise of the middle class, higher wages and better conditions for the workers who were left, an increased reliance on scientific explanations for natural phenomena, and therefore a growing distrust of religion. "The biomedical catastrophe took away charisma from kings, eroded popular support for their veneration and self-esteem as God's anointed and as war leaders and money providers," writes Norman F. Cantor in *In the Wake of the Plague*. In England, "it drove a sensitive, intelligent monarch like Richard II toward anguished behavior and antisocial, politically imprudent policy that led the nobility headed by his cousin to bring him down and kill him."

In *An Irish History of Civilization*, Don Akenson writes about "black plague syndrome," the consequences to a society of living through a major pandemic. Akenson tells the story of Dr. Peter Buck, director of Maori Hygiene in New Zealand in the 1920s, who found that "the after-shocks of the massive 1918 influenza epidemic... had fallen most heavily on the Maori." These included "a fanatical chasing after religious explanations by some, denial of the existing god by others, personal guilt for having survived, false gaiety, gaping holes in the social hierarchy, desperate attempts to shore up the social pyramid, violent arguments about social status, inheritance, property, debts and dues." Six years later, he found similar aftershocks on Western Samoa, where the speed and mortality of the epidemic had been greater than recorded anywhere else in the world. Māori society had been transformed by disaster from one of peaceful, communal living to one that resembled Western culture.

Contemporary historians warn of similar repercussions from Covid-19. In *Apollo's Arrow*, Nicholas A. Christakis sees the widening gap between Democrats and Republicans and the resurgence of rampant racism as a direct result of America's experience with the crisis. Just as Jews were blamed for the Black Death, and Spaniards for the recurrence of the plague in 1630 and again for the 1918 influenza pandemic, Americans gave in to "the temptation to blame others, typically outsiders or minorities, for calamity in a time of plague." In the 1940s and 1950s, families of polio victims were shunned and even run out of some towns. "This kind of fearful and dehumanizing thinking can also find expression in the seemingly reasonable desire to close borders, identifying 'outsiders' as the source of a problem," turning America into an "us and them" society that will have long-lasting effects.

This division into us-and-them has happened elsewhere, as well: Canadian psychologists Nigel Mantou Lou and Kimberly Noels point to "data from the Vancouver Police Department [showing] a 717 percent increase of reports of hate crimes targeting Asian Canadians in 2020 compared to the previous year."

In the April 2021 issue of *Harper's*, Elliot Ackerman, in an article titled "Civil Warning," compares post-pandemic America to the United States in the years leading up to the Civil War, arguing that the gathering of forces during the pandemic chillingly echoes the bipartisan rhetoric of the 1850s. "Although today's geographic divisions are not quite as stark as the divisions between free and slave states in the nineteenth century," he writes, "geography matters less in our atomized and hyperconnected society." Anger and discontent travel fast on social media, and—as seen in Washington, D.C., on January 6, 2021—violence can be organized in minutes.

Elise Labott, writing in *Foreign Policy* on July 22, 2021, notes similar disruptions in countries around the world. "From Cuba to South Africa to Colombia to Haiti," she writes, violent protests have erupted against "preexisting social, economic, and political hardships, which fallout from the Covid-19 pandemic only inflamed further." She warns that these uprisings are "merely a foreshadowing of the post-coronavirus global tinderbox that's looming as existing tensions in countries across the world morph into broader civil unrest."

Although there may be an After Times for the pandemic, SARS-COV-2, the coronavirus that causes it, will probably remain among us, possibly forever.

Christakis proposes that the coronavirus OC43, one of the four that causes the common cold, began life as the coronavirus responsible for the Russian flu, a pandemic that swept through Europe in 1889–90, killing 250,000 people. OC43 originated as a highly contagious respiratory disease of cattle but in the 1880s separated from its bovine reservoir. As it evolved (by variant-producing mutations), it became weaker—which means smarter, since killing one's host is not a good survival strategy for anything. A virus needs a host in order to reproduce.

"After being among us for a century," Christakis writes, "this virus would have further evolved to be a mild pathogen that just causes the common cold today." The bird flu outbreak of 2005 flared up and died out quickly because it quickly killed such a large percentage of its hosts that it didn't leave itself time to evolve into a milder infection. Covid-19 has taken that time, and it is likely that future occurrences of the disease will be mild enough—like the common cold is now—to allow its hosts to continue to circulate and spread the virus to other hosts. The virus will then live to pass on its genetic material to future generations, the sole aim of evolution. It's almost as though Christakis predicted Omicron.

Covid-19 may take that evolutionary path to perpetual survival—or we might. Rupert Beale, a clinician scientist at the Francis Crick Institute in London, England—"a biomedical research institute working...

to make discoveries about how life works"—noted
that, over time, humans may develop a kind of "memory immunity" to the coronavirus. Those who have
had Covid-19 or have been vaccinated, he writes in the
London Review of Books (March 4, 2021), "may get
infected again, but because they have some measure
of immunity their infections will be mild." Some of us
will need a booster shot now and then, he says, perhaps
every two years, as "seasonal coronaviruses tend to
rise in two-yearly cycles."

In one form or another, Covid will be with us well
into the After Times, which in effect means there will
be no After Times. "There will be people living with
the impact of Covid long after the pandemic is over,"
Craig Spencer, of the NewYork-Presbyterian/Colum-
bia University Irving Medical Center, told *The Atlantic*
in April 2021. "This is not made up or in the minds of
people who are sickly. This is real."

The pandemic could provide us with an opportunity
to learn from our mistakes. Although it feels wrong to
look for benefits from a disaster that has killed more
than 15 million people—like politicians who talk about
the benefits of climate change—the pandemic has the
potential to change many things that needed changing. Speaking of climate change, the world burned less
fossil fuel during the pandemic; air pollution levels
in twenty countries dropped 20 percent in 2020, and
carbon dioxide emissions fell by 6.4 percent (thanks
largely to reduced emissions from aviation, which fell

48 percent below their 2019 level) both on the ground and in the troposphere. As restrictions on travel were lifted in late 2021, those figures jumped back to almost pre-pandemic levels, but there is a lesson in there somewhere if we choose to learn it.

During the pandemic and the resulting slump in international shipping, the oceans became quieter. For the first time in decades, dolphins and whales were able to hear each other and could socialize and navigate as they had during the era of sail, when Darwin declared that the thought processes of dolphins and humans were hardly dissimilar. Modern oceanographers declared 2020 "the year of the quiet ocean." Like Covid-19, the silence started in the coastal areas around China and gradually spread to the rest of the seven seas. The noise rose sharply again in 2021 as normal freighter traffic resumed.

Another lesson we might take from the pandemic is that women are better at managing countries than men. As reported in *The Guardian* in August 2020, the countries led by women handled the crisis and fared much better than countries run by men. New Zealand (Jacinda Ardern), Germany (Angela Merkel), Finland (Sanna Marin), Iceland (Katrín Jakobsdóttir), and Taiwan (Tsai Ing-wen) all kept their Covid numbers down and managed to get through the early stages of the pandemic, at least, in relatively good economic shape. The countries with the worst Covid records— the US (Donald Trump), the UK (Boris Johnson), Brazil

(Jair Bolsonaro), India (Narendra Modi), and Venezuela (Nicolás Maduro)—were all headed by men, and men who tended politically to the far right.

In *A Paradise Built in Hell*, Rebecca Solnit recounts that after the Halifax Explosion of 1917, St. Paul's Anglican Church, situated close to the devastated harbor, served as a refuge for 350 survivors of the cataclysm that had destroyed half the city. Two years later, the curate of that church, Samuel Henry Prince, went to Columbia University in New York and began writing what became his doctoral dissertation, *Catastrophe and Social Change*, a book that became the foundation document for the study of the aftermath of disasters.

"Its premise," writes Solnit, "is that disaster begets social and political change... That is, disasters open up societies to change, accelerate change that was under way, or break the hold of whatever was preventing change." It was Prince who defined "civil society" as "a new sense of unity in dealing with common problems." Part of the impetus in working toward a civil society is a sudden realization, illuminated by the disaster, that governments cannot be depended on to solve the problems created by the disaster.

Solnit gives many examples: after the massive earthquake that shook Mexico City in 1985, when thousands of people were trapped under collapsed factories and poorly built apartment buildings, the mayor sent the army out, not to rescue those trapped in the rubble, but to prevent looters from entering the damaged buildings and stealing the factory- and store-owners' goods and equipment. Thousands died who could have been rescued. In the aftermath of the earthquake, citizens' groups formed to organize workers and families to oust corrupt officials and organize housing rights committees—and the country's first women-led union. These movements were, writes Solnit, " 'the moral center' of the earthquake, or rather of the society galvanized by that earthquake. Support came from all over."

The pandemic has had more widely distributed shocks to our system than the Mexican earthquake. It has been a truly global phenomenon, more like climate change, except that we do not get daily reports on climate change in every country in every part of the world. Perhaps we should. Perhaps we will. It's encouraging that in the midst of a global pandemic, 197 national groups met in Glasgow for a two-week summit on climate change, the United Nations' COP26. Covid has made us more conscious than ever of the plight of the other, the hardships and loneliness suffered in (to us) remote corners of the globe, and of the necessity of addressing global problems with a united voice.

"While being enormously disruptive and painful," writes astrobiologist Lewis Dartnell, "crises also invariably nurture the emergence of great common purpose, solidarity, creativity, and improvisation." Positive changes, such as renewed political action to mitigate climate change, international cooperation in confronting other common threats, and more determined efforts to create a truly civil society, could become the "moral center" of the Covid-19 pandemic.

The one thing we know for certain is that the world is not going back to the way it was in the Before Times. It's up to us what shape it takes in the After Times.

Acknowledgments

WITHIN MY OWN FAMILY, I was part of a microcosm from which I could observe and participate in the wider pandemic. Of fifteen family members, including our children and their spouses, our grandchildren and their partners, ten contracted Covid-19 (two of them twice), two were immunocompromised by comorbidities, twelve were double-vaxxed, five were triple-vaxxed, and one was quadruple-vaxxed. Three of the adults were unvaccinated—one for ideological reasons, one because of comorbidity, and one because they weren't convinced they needed to be. Two were caregivers to the two who were vulnerable, four were under the age of twelve, and two were vaccinated when their workplaces required it. As a result, I was able to experience at close range the effects of society at-large of living through the pandemic, and that helped make me more sympathetic to experiences I might not have had otherwise. Although this book isn't about them, I certainly couldn't have written it without them.

Earlier versions of eight of the entries in this lexicon first appeared in *Queen's Quarterly*. I am grateful to the journal's editor, James Carson, with whom I corresponded while he was stranded by the pandemic in Australia, and to the journal's production editor in Kingston, Steve Anderson, who over the years has massaged more than a dozen of my essays, stories, and even a poem onto its pages. I am also hugely indebted to Dr. David Walker, professor and former dean of medicine at Queen's University, who read the excerpt and then this manuscript and made many valuable suggestions.

Many friends shared their Covid experiences with me as I was working on the book. In particular, I am grateful to Pam Cross, Jamie Swift, Andrew Nikiforuk, and John Harriss, all of whom have written about Covid and contributed their individual perspectives to my own thinking. I have also enjoyed comparing notes with my friends David Homel in Montreal, Pedro Serrano in Mexico City, and Christopher Hixson, Mitchell Kahan, Jennifer Clement, Lena Bartula, and Judith Gill in San Miguel de Allende during our many conversations in Canada and Mexico.

My agent, Martha Webb, gave me valuable advice and support as the book neared what, in the context of the pandemic, had to pass for completion. My friend Rob Sanders, founder of Greystone Books, was his usual enthusiastic self when I sent him the early draft, and Nancy Flight added much-needed touches of accuracy and grace to the manuscript. A book covering three years of breaking news requires constant updating, fact-checking, and citation juggling, and James Penco was sensitive and diligent in keeping my observations accurate and on point.

And, of course, my wife, Merilyn Simonds, made me feel, as she always does, that this writing game is worth the candle. I am forever thankful that she and I are a bubble.

Index of Terms